Now Wh....

What to Expect in Your First Year of Bariatric Surgery

Geof Shuford

Now What? What to expect from your first year of bariatric surgery

Cover design and artwork: Robin Locke Monda

ISBN: 979-8-9898353-0-0

Printed in the United States of America

This book is dedicated to all the people over the years that have helped me grow and learn. Without this I would not be able to share my knowledge with others.

I'd like specifically thank Stephanie Preston and Todd Weber for all their support with this book, as well as my editor for all their work on making this a better book.

Contents

Introduction

What You Can Expect from This Book

As a personal trainer and bariatric mindset coach who has been helping bariatric patients for more than ten years, I wrote this book because I want to offer bariatric patients a path that can help them establish a successful weight-loss journey, starting at the very beginning of the process and proceeding through the first year of the journey, with a brief look at the years ahead. This book looks at some of the more common setbacks to make you aware of possible obstacles in your path—and be prepared to meet them. You may not encounter all these (temporary) roadblocks, and it's possible that not all the suggestions will work for you, but I hope you find enough good information that you feel like you know what to do once you're no longer under medical supervision.

It's my goal to give you a good view of what it takes to be successful in all parts of your weight loss without having to do hours of research. But it's important to note that individual problems always come up, and these unique circumstances are beyond the scope of this book. While I do my best to be accurate on common suggestions and recommendations, there may be some disparity between what I've written and what your surgical team asks of you. If you run up against this, your surgeon's advice will always supersede whatever is written here. But despite these individual issues, there are many parts of bariatric surgery that almost everyone experiences—and that's where this advice can help set you up for success.

To be successful, it's imperative that you understand from the beginning that this isn't something that can be done quickly; it will take many months and more than likely many years to see all the positives. Don't expect a quick route to your weight-loss destination: after all, it's called a weight-loss *journey*, not a trip.

Why Is This Weight Loss Referred to as a Journey?

Think about it for a second. A trip is a one-time adventure that comes and goes. It may change you a little bit or for a little while, or you may forget about it altogether. A journey, on the other hand, has twists and turns and encompasses a long stretch of time. It is often associated with the different phases of your life. High school, the college years, building an intimate partnership, and forming a family: we think of these phases in terms of the substantial change they bring to our lives, transforming us in considerable and lasting ways. When you think of it in these terms, weight-loss surgery seems more like a journey than a trip. Like marriage or college, this procedure will profoundly affect your life. It's worth the efforts I'll suggest.

Any successful journey has a preparation phase, an embarkation phase, and then the travel itself. It's no different with weight-loss surgery. Your preparation phase: planning around the right surgical and support team, getting your home ready, and doing some mental prep for the journey ahead. Then you'll embark with the surgery itself, and the journey truly starts when you are wheeled into the recovery room. And it doesn't stop there. You'll continue to adapt to the changes and learn how to manage your weight for years to come. You might find that there's no single destination—maybe you'll find new goals and things you want to try. The journey may be long, but it can be rewarding.

Like any journey, the bariatric weight-loss journey starts out exciting, a new and unknown adventure. This can be scary, with new pains, some elevated anxiety, and maybe even some doubt about why you started the journey in the first place. Yet there are some amazing new things that will happen to you quickly: these can include the reduction or cessation of medication, better sleep, and reduced joint pain, all of which help build your motivation. This period of high motivation, known as the honeymoon phase, doesn't last forever, though, and you may find that old habits and desires will start to creep back into your life. Though you'll be early in the process, knowing what lies ahead will help you plan for periods of low motivation and prevent you from letting these dips turn into a detour to the journey known as an "expansion phase." This expansion phase has two meanings. One refers to a time during which you expand your menu choices to include foods and drinks that do not support your weight-loss or maintenance goals. Foods like ice cream, chocolate, soda, and simple carbs (such as bread, crackers, and potato chips) can sabotage your transformation. You can have those—in moderation. But you want to prevent these foods from creeping back into your daily life and completely derailing your journey.

The other meaning of "expansion phase" is more literal. You will very likely gain some weight at some point in your journey. It happens. This expansion is well known in the bariatric community, and it's often referred to as the "rebound phase." It typically happens about three to five years after surgery. It's nothing to be worried about, but you should be aware of it, understand that it can happen, and remember that it's normal—and in all likelihood, you'll be doing fine. Along with knowing about the expansion phase, another important issue will be how your relationships with yourself and other people will change. There will be people in your life who will not like the path you have taken. They may belittle you and your decision and try to minimize your accomplishments. You may be surprised about who these people turn out to be. You will have to minimize their voices and remember why you're taking the journey and what your goals are. There will also be people in your life who will provide you with immense support. These are the people and relationships that you need to seek out and foster. You won't need too many people in your corner but having at least a few strong supporters will make a significant impact on your weight loss. And finally, to make this weight-loss journey as successful as you can, there will need to be a change to the relationship you have with yourself. This is the relationship that is the most important to grow and make stronger. This book gives you lots of examples and information to help with this.

At some point on this journey, you will find yourself in the maintenance phase. This is when you have reached your weight-loss goals (or gotten close) and your health and habits have changed for the better. It's a time when the new habits talked about in this book become part of your daily routine. It's when you see yourself as the healthy, active person you've become and more. The maintenance phase is when you both maintain the success you've achieved and start to branch out into new parts of your life. While it can feel that once you've reached this part of the journey you've made it—and in some respects you have—this is a dynamic stage and could easily be seen as the start of a completely new life journey. While I've outlined the general stages of this journey, understand that this isn't a linear process. It will take time, you will fumble through parts, you will seek comfort in old habits and thinking, and that is normal and expected. These are not failures; as long as you are still trusting in yourself, you will see success.

What Is Success?

You'll notice that I have used the phrase "to be successful with your bariatric surgery" throughout this book. So, what does "being successful" mean? The obvious answer is a loss of your excess body fat. Although that's one answer, it's not a full answer. There's more to this journey than just losing body fat. Bariatric surgery gives you a tool that, if used correctly, provides you with a jump-start on building a new, healthy life. Think beyond the process of losing the excess body fat to what that loss will enable you to do. You'll be able to move easier, you'll be more active, you'll sleep better, you'll have increased confidence, and so much more! If you embrace these parts of the weight-loss process, "success" becomes much more than just losing the weight. "Success" starts to encompass what you can now do with your transformed body. "Success" is about a new life. My hope for you is that this book will help you get the most out of your journey, that it will help you avoid or minimize the pitfalls that come along with this new life. I hope you'll refer to these pages as a guide to building the life you want.

Why Is This Procedure Called a Tool?

You may be wondering what I was talking about in the previous section when I referred to bariatric surgery giving you a tool. If you have talked to anyone about bariatric surgery or read any other parts of this book, you will see and hear this procedure being called a tool, because that's what it is. A tool is anything that helps make a task easier. A hammer is a tool that makes driving nails into wood easier, a car is a tool that makes traveling places easier, a dumbbell is a tool that makes getting stronger easier. Bariatric surgery is a tool that makes losing a significant amount of weight easier.

As with any tool, there is a learning process for how to use it effectively and safely. That has to do with how well you understand what the tool is built to do. With bariatric surgery, the tool is built to limit the number of calories you can take in, and for that to be effective, you have to know how to use it correctly. The rules of the tool, discussed in chapter 4, give you a great starting point on using this tool the right way. Whether you use it correctly depends on how well you can modify strongly held habits. This book will touch on some of the more common habit pitfalls in the mindset sections.

What Bariatric Surgery Is (and Isn't)

Before going any further on what bariatric surgery is and how it works, I want to talk about what it is not. This procedure is not a cheat. I'm bringing this topic up at the beginning of this book because it's a statement that is made frequently. Or it's hidden in a question that implies it's "taking the easy way out" or that you "cheated."

But what are you cheating? Who are you cheating? When you cheat, you're breaking the rules—and what are the rules for weight loss? Fundamentally, there is only one rule to weight loss: create a consistent calorie deficit. Weight-loss surgery isn't cheating, and it's not a shortcut. Creating a calorie deficit is the main purpose of bariatric surgery. I want to debunk this notion that bariatric surgery is cheating.

Obesity isn't something that you give yourself; it is something that you have. We all know a person who eats terribly, never exercises, and still somehow maintains an "ideal" weight. Their genetics and metabolism support a slender physique. (This doesn't mean that they are inherently healthy—a bad diet and lack of exercise will eventually catch up with them, though it may not be through weight gain.) You, unfortunately, have the genetics, the metabolism, and quite possibly a mental state that promotes excessive weight gain.

Your weight loss has never been as easy as "eat less and exercise" implies. But you've probably tried that. In fact, you've likely tried it all: personal trainers, group classes, spin classes, every diet under the sun, counting "points" and calories, new fitness equipment, shakes, and prepackaged meals. And yet, you are still at a weight you don't like and that isn't healthy for you. If "eat less and exercise" is the rule you're supposed to follow, you did! You played by the rules and ended up no better than before (or in some cases, even heavier and unhealthier).

Let's take a different tack with this and say you didn't exhaust all your other options before weight-loss surgery. Then bariatric surgery is cheating, right?

Nope.

Again, the basic purpose of weight-loss surgery is all about limiting your calorie intake so you will lose weight (though there are many other positive aspects like reducing the risk of death by 40 percent.[1]) Weight-loss surgery is simply one form of every other legitimate weight-loss program out there. It's more aggressive than counting points or going on the keto diet, but its purpose is no different: to help you lose weight and build a healthier life.

In many ways, weight-loss surgery is a more effective weight-loss program than a lot of the other ones you've tried. It can improve type 2 diabetes, kidney disease, and quality of life. It's also a procedure that you can't easily give up on. Yet bariatric surgery requires some hard work and lifestyle changes, and if you don't implement these things, you can completely fail at losing weight (which is the reason I wrote this book.) As with any other program, if it's going to succeed, you have to work at it.

Maybe bariatric surgery is cheating because it's too fast and easy?

With bariatric surgery, it's not out of the ordinary to lose 70-plus pounds in less than a year with no "real work" on your part. You won't see this very often in other legitimate weight-loss programs. That still doesn't mean bariatric surgery is cheating or wrong; it's just different. You have a tool that allows weight loss to occur faster than usual (for a limited time). And instead of thinking of the speed of weight loss as a shortcut or a cheat, think of it as a jump-start to being able to do what you want.

Anyone who has been successful at losing weight and keeping it off with bariatric surgery knows that it requires a lot of work and dedication, much more than just a few cardio sessions a week or "mostly" eating right. This procedure doesn't give you a free pass from eating right and exercising. If you're going to be successful long-term, those have to be a part of your overall plan. Yet these things become easier and more enjoyable once you have shed a significant amount of weight.

Bariatric surgery gets you quickly to the point where moving becomes easier, and because you are healthier, you can do the work more effectively. While before the surgery movement was difficult, now it's not. You are freer to be more active. This is one of the biggest differences with weight-loss surgery compared with other forms of weight loss. Traditional weight-loss efforts are slow to get you to a point where you can do more things easier. If you can get over the hump of losing a significant percentage of your excess body fat, you are positioned to continue with the weight loss in a much more pain-free and healthier state. That is an assist, not a cheat.

8

Bariatric surgery is a tool. Sure, it's drastic by design, but there is nothing illegitimate about it. When you hear people call it a cheat, understand that they don't know what weight-loss surgery really takes. You can help them understand if you like, or you can just let it roll off your back and know that you are just as dedicated as any other person on the weight-loss journey—if not more so.

SECTION 1: The Tool and the Surgeon

Chapter 1: Different Tools for Different Needs

Bariatric surgery is the modification of your stomach and possibly part of your small intestines with the goal of helping you lose weight (and improve your overall health) by restricting the size of your stomach and possibly reducing the amount of nutrients your body can absorb.

There are a few types of tools (procedures) used to achieve this weight loss, and each has specific pros and cons. In this chapter I will go over some of the more common types of surgeries and the typical population that each one is designed to assist. The descriptions of these different procedures should help you when you talk with your surgeon about which one is best for you.

But before going further with the different types of surgeries, let's talk about how your digestive system works before any modifications are made. It may seem a little long and at times a little gross, but because different surgery types affect different organs and parts of the digestive process, it's important to know what will happen. This can help you visualize how the different procedures affect the digestive system and how each modification helps you lose weight.

Your Plumbing and How It Keeps You Alive

Believe it or not, digestion starts with your nose. When a smell hits your brain, it signals your salivary glands to start producing saliva in your mouth. Saliva helps moisten your food and begins the digestive process by secreting enzymes to start breaking down carbohydrates and fats. In addition, the process of chewing breaks down the food to reduce the amount of work the stomach must do. Once the food is broken down enough by the enzymes and chewing, it is pushed through your esophagus and down to your stomach, where the main process of digestion occurs. At this point the chewed food is called bolus.

In this stage, two methods, mechanical and chemical, work together to further break down your food. First, the mechanical: The stomach is made up of smooth muscle tissue and a lining full of wrinkles called rugae, or gastric folds. These two parts of the stomach combine to help break down the bolus.

The smooth muscle tissue contracts and relaxes in a process called peristalsis to mix the bolus with the strong acid that is secreted in the stomach, allowing for a more complete breakdown of the food. Additionally, the rugae assist this process by having places where the bolus can be gripped, making churning of the food easier.

The second method of digestion is the chemical, or enzymatic, process. The innermost layer of the stomach is lined with small pores that secrete mucus, hydrochloric acid, and digestive enzymes. Once food enters your stomach, the stomach secretes these juices. Each has a different purpose. Mucus will start to spread along the inner walls of the stomach to protect the lining from the very strong acid as well as from the digestive enzymes. The hydrochloric acid and enzymes enter the main stomach pouch to break down proteins and fats. This process takes between one and two hours and creates a paste called chyme. At this point the peristalsis helps move this chyme into the small intestines through an opening at the base of the stomach called the pyloric sphincter. This sphincter separates the first part of the small intestine, aka the duodenum, from the stomach. The final process of digestion takes place in the duodenum.

Within the duodenum, different enzymes, which are secreted from the liver and gallbladder, continue the breakdown of the chyme into its most basic elements. Fats are converted into fatty acids, proteins turn into more basic amino acids, and carbohydrates become different polysaccharides (sugars). In addition, the duodenum's mucus walls neutralize the acid that is mixed in with the chyme, protecting the remaining sections of the small and large intestines.

Entering the rest of the small intestine, these nutrients and minerals are pressed against fingerlike projections known as villi, which absorb them into the bloodstream. This is also the final stage in the digestion of carbohydrates, when enzymes in the small intestines break down the polysaccharides into their final forms (glucose, fructose, and galactose), where they are taken up into the bloodstream. This process of nutrient and mineral absorption takes several hours to complete. The small intestine connects to the base of the large intestine, and whatever matter hasn't been absorbed is moved through as waste.

The large intestine is also home to a large host of bacteria that have a multitude of beneficial effects on the body. This bacteria lives off the fiber and nondigestible parts of the foods you eat.

Until it enters the small intestine, the food is not a part of the body; it is just being broken down to be absorbed later. It is only when this "food" enters the small intestine that the sugars, amino acids, and fats get distributed into the rest of the body. The longer this substance moves through the small intestine, the more is absorbed.

As this description shows, digestion requires a lot of steps, each occurring in a different part of the digestive tract. Bariatric surgery changes parts of your digestive tract, and those changes alter how your body absorbs foods and nutrients. The type of surgery you and your surgeon choose will change how your body works.

How Does This Digestive Process Change with the Different Forms of Bariatric Surgery?

Each of the procedures that follow has its pros and cons. Because some procedures are aggressive, they will only be available to you if you meet certain criteria and don't have existing comorbidities. This section gives you a good overview of how each procedure works to help you lose excess body fat. You will need to discuss in detail with your surgeon and primary care physician which of these (or some other form of weight loss) will work best for you.

Roux-en-Y Bypass or Gastric Bypass (RNY)

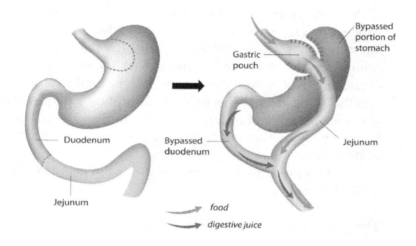

Gastric pouch

Bypassed portion of stomach

Duodenum

Bypassed duodenum

Jejunum

Jejunum

food

digestive juice

The Roux-en-Y gastric bypass relies on malabsorption and restriction. It gets its name from the way the upper small intestine is rerouted, creating a "Y" shape (it is also why it's called a gastric "bypass"). The procedure has two main parts: First, a small "pouch" is created in the upper part of the stomach, just below the esophagus. This pouch is created by cutting away the lower, larger portion of the stomach. The incisions are stapled closed, creating a new, much more restrictive pouch. The remaining stomach stays in place, and the gastric juices still play a part in the digestive/absorption phase, just farther down in the small intestines.

The second part of the bypass cuts the small intestine 40 to 75 centimeters (16 to 30 inches) below the stomach's pyloric sphincter, bypassing the duodenum. The small intestine is rerouted up to the newly created stomach pouch. The 40-to-75-centimeter section of small intestine and duodenum is then attached farther down on the small intestine.

As a result of this change, the chyme that comes out of the stomach pouch skips the digestive enzymes in the duodenum, effectively making it difficult for the small intestine to absorb any nutrients. Only after those 40 to 75 centimeters, when the chyme meets back up with the duodenum, is it broken down enough to be readily absorbed into the bloodstream. This delayed absorption's purpose is to reduce the amount of fat, sugar, and amino acids taken into the body, in turn giving the body less energy it needs to store as fat.

This procedure is usually restricted to people with a BMI of 35 or greater.

The good stuff about this procedure:

- Reduces the amount of food you can eat.
- Shortens the amount of time food spends in the small intestine so there's less absorption of calories.
- Lowers the amount of the hunger hormone ghrelin released, due to a reduction in stomach size.
- Removes or reduces the symptoms of GERD, or gastroesophageal reflux disease.

The bad stuff about this procedure:

- High risk of vitamin malnutrition.
- High risk of calcium deficiency.
- Increased risk of gallstones due to the rapid weight loss.
- Higher risk of dumping. (chapter 7)

16

Mini Gastric Bypass

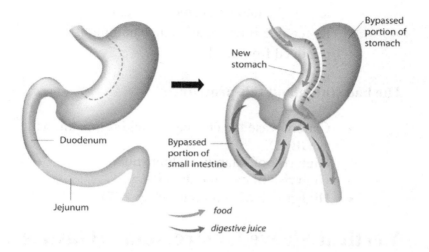

New stomach

Bypassed portion of stomach

Duodenum

Bypassed portion of small intestine

Jejunum

food

digestive juice

The mini gastric bypass works very similarly to the standard bypass, but it's a slightly less complex procedure. This surgery cuts a small pouch from the stomach and attaches part of the intestines a few feet past the duodenum. This bypass of the duodenum reduces absorption of calories because the chyme mixes with the enzymes from the gallbladder and liver farther down the small intestines. Because the small intestine is attached closer to the stomach, less work needs to be done. In most ways the mini gastric bypass is very similar to the standard Roux-en Y gastric bypass in how it works to help you lose weight.

The good stuff about this procedure:

- A faster and easier surgery for your surgeon

17

- Food spends less time in the small intestine for less absorption of calories.
- Reduction in stomach size means you'll have less of the hunger hormone ghrelin.
- Reversible if necessary, since nothing is removed from the body.

The bad stuff about this procedure:

- Can increase the chances of acid reflux known as GERD.
- High risk of vitamin malnutrition.
- High risk of calcium deficiency.
- Higher risk of dumping. (chapter 7)

Vertical Sleeve Gastrectomy (Gastric Sleeve)

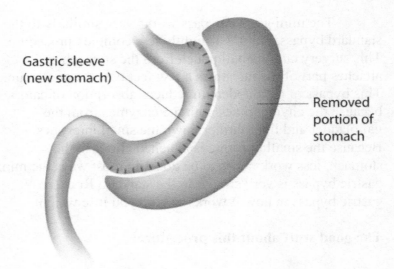

Gastric sleeve (new stomach)

Removed portion of stomach

Copyright Alila Medical Media

Where the duodenal switch and Roux-en-Y work with both food restriction and malabsorption of the food, the gastric sleeve, also called vertical sleeve gastrectomy, uses only restriction to help you lose excess body fat. In this procedure, the surgeon removes between 70 and 80 percent of your stomach, preserving the upper, or esophageal, portion, where the food enters your stomach, and the lower, or pyloric/duodenal portion of the stomach. The incision and staple line follow the curvature of the stomach, leaving a banana-shaped pouch. Unlike the bypass, with this procedure the section of the stomach that was cut off is removed from the body.

This smaller stomach reduces the amount of food you can eat by signaling the brain more quickly than your full-size stomach that you are full. The remaining portion of your digestive system stays intact, reducing the chance for malabsorption of nutrients.

This procedure is typically suggested to patients with a BMI in the 30 to 40 range and who have fewer comorbidities due to their obesity.

The good stuff about this procedure:

- Reduces the amount of food you can eat at one time.
- Less chance of dumping because the pyloric sphincter remains intact.
- Less limitations on medication and multivitamin pill sizes.
- No significant malabsorption of nutrients.
- Reduction in stomach size means less of the hunger hormone ghrelin.

The bad stuff about this procedure:

- There is no chance for a reversal.
- Higher chance of gallstones.
- Can continue or increase your symptoms of GERD.

Duodenal Switch

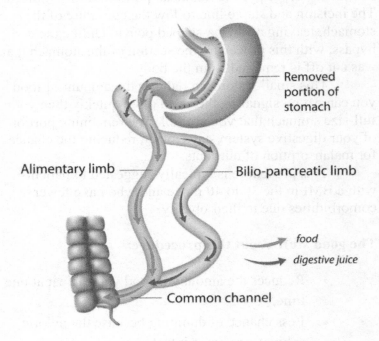

Removed portion of stomach

Alimentary limb

Bilio-pancreatic limb

food

digestive juice

Common channel

The duodenal switch is named after the first part of the small intestine, called the duodenum. It's where bile is secreted from the gallbladder and liver to break down the chyme into the components of the foods (amino acids, sugars, and fatty acids). These components are then passed into the remaining small intestine, where they are absorbed into the bloodstream.

This procedure relocates the duodenum about three-quarters of the way down the small intestine, so it's no longer at the head of the small intestine. The bypassed portion of the small intestine becomes the pathway for the digestive juices that come from the gallbladder and liver. The new top portion of the small intestine is then attached directly to the stomach pouch. Due to this, the chyme that comes out of the stomach initially avoids the bile from the gallbladder and liver. The chyme is pushed through the small intestine and bypasses the absorption phase. Only when the chyme mixes with the enzyme secreted from the duodenum farther down the small intestine does the food get broken down enough to be absorbed. Because the chyme spends a limited time in the small intestines, fewer fats, sugars, and amino acids are absorbed by the body. Because fewer nutrients are absorbed, the body has less energy (calories) to store.

This procedure also removes a large section of your stomach, restricting the amount of food you will be able to eat in one sitting. Because this procedure preserves the pyloric sphincter, the lower part of your stomach that controls the release of the chyme into the small intestine, the risk of a side effect called dumping (see chapter 7) is smaller than with the gastric bypass.

This procedure is usually restricted to people who have a BMI of 45 or greater.

The good stuff about this procedure:

- Reduces the amount of food you can eat.
- Keeps dumping syndrome under control.
- Food has less time in the small intestine for less absorption of calories.

- Reduces stomach size so you'll have less of the hunger hormone ghrelin.
- Results in higher weight loss than any other procedure.

The bad stuff about this procedure:

- High risk of vitamin malnutrition, especially with fat-soluble vitamins A, D, E, and K.
- High risk of protein malnutrition.
- High risk of calcium deficiency.
- Increased risk of gallstones due to the rapid weight loss.
- Less absorption of fats, which can lead to smelly flatulence and diarrhea.

Adjustable Gastric Band (Lap Band)

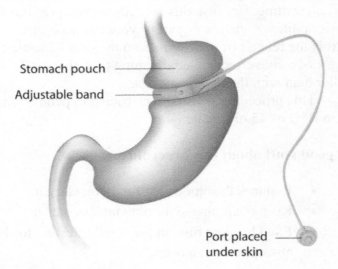

Stomach pouch

Adjustable band

Port placed under skin

22

Most surgeons have stopped using this procedure due to its higher failure rate—that is, most people don't lose weight and maintain that loss with the band.

Gastric banding is a process that surgically adds a silicone band around the upper portion of the stomach to restrict the amount of food that can be eaten. Like other forms of bariatric surgery, this restriction results in a smaller pouch that signals the brain that it is full more quickly than a nonmodified stomach. The band is connected to a port that is placed under the skin near your abdomen. This port is used to add or remove saline, which changes the amount of restriction on your stomach, which in turn changes how much food you can eat in one sitting.

As with the gastric sleeve, this procedure is suggested to patients with a BMI in the 30 to 40 range and who have fewer comorbidities due to their obesity.

The good stuff about this procedure:

- No permanent modification to your internal organs.
- Restricts your food intake.
- An easier surgery than other forms of bariatric surgery.
- No dumping syndrome.

The bad stuff about this procedure:

- Overall, less-effective weight loss than other forms of bariatric surgery.
- Band slippage, making it less effective.
- Higher chance of weight regain because your hunger hormone isn't affected by this surgery.

Now that you have a basic understanding of what different types of surgery are available, the next step is finding the right surgeon, learning how to deal with insurance or self-pay, and going out of the country for your surgery.

Chapter 2: Finding Your Surgeon, How to Pay, and How to Prep for Your Surgery

There are many steps you will need to take while you're preparing for your surgery: finding the right surgeon, investigating insurance coverage, and moving through all the tests and doctors' appointments you will need, to name a few. As thorough as your surgical team and insurance company may be, they aren't able to cover *everything* for your unique situation. You'll need to sit down and do some planning on your own. This section will help guide you through this process.

How Are You Going to Pay for Your Surgery?

One of the first things you should do as you investigate this surgery is to decide how you are going to pay for it. Will you be going through your insurance, or will you be paying for the procedure from your own pocket (aka self-pay)? These decisions will affect many other options that are available to you.

Self-pay

If you take the self-pay route, you are on the hook for the entire cost of the surgery—but taking this path allows you to bypass some of the requirements that most insurance companies impose. The biggest is increasing your pool of surgeons that you can choose from. You may also be scheduled for the surgery much quicker than with insurance. Yet there are still requirements you will have to meet to be scheduled for the surgery.

- Your primary care doctor must clear you for the surgery (as may other doctors if you have comorbid conditions).
- You'll need to have current lab work.
- You'll need a consultation with your surgeon of choice.
- You'll likely want a consultation with a registered dietitian.
- You'll be asked to have a psychiatric evaluation.
- You'll need to get a clearance regarding your cardiac health.
- You will need a clear understanding of what's involved with the surgery and the aftercare and a willingness to do the work it takes to make you successful.

If you are unable to pay for this surgery in one lump sum and your insurance will not cover the procedure for you, talk with your surgeon's office about a surgical loan. In some cases, the surgeon's practice can help limit the upfront cost of the surgery and allow you to pay in installments. This option may not be available with all surgeons, so as you are interviewing potential specialists for this procedure, ask if this is an option they offer. If you can self-pay up front, some surgeons may offer a discount. If you're considering self-pay, also ask if the surgeon's office offers a package deal. This could include some or all of the presurgical requirements like lab and blood work, psychiatric evaluation, hospital fees, and other fees. If your surgeon offers this option, ask if the package entails any limitations around your choice of specialists, such as your psychiatrist or lab work providers.

Another issue to ask prospective surgeons about if you're planning to self-pay is coverage for surgical complications. It's nearly impossible to predict whether you'll experience any or what they might be. So, it's important to ask if your surgeon will cover complications in their initial fee or if you will be on the hook for any extra work that needs to be done due to these unforeseen complications. Not only does this help with budgeting, but it will also make dealing with the complications easier, if they should arise.

Insurance

If you intend to use insurance to help offset the cost of bariatric surgery, your first step has to be contacting your insurer. You'll want to get information on how much of the procedure is covered and how much out-of-pocket cost you should expect. You should also request a list of doctors and hospitals your insurance has in its network so that when you start looking for a doctor, there are no surprises. Do not assume coverage is the same for one insurance company. Employer-sponsored plans may include or exclude specific procedures, so what's covered for insurance companies will differ accordingly.

One piece of information that can help you when discussing options and pricing around this surgery are the billing codes. These are universal codes used by doctors, hospitals, and insurance companies to know how much to charge for different procedures. While they don't typically come up when you are investigating different procedures, having them on hand can help you when you are discussing the procedure with your doctor's billing office or your insurance company. They are typically easy to find by going online and searching terms such as "weight loss surgery billing codes," "bariatric surgery billing codes," or the name of the procedure you are planning on getting plus "billing codes."

In addition to investigating the coverage and out-of-pocket expenses for the surgery itself, ask if any or all of the necessary pre-op work and tests you will need are covered. You'll need to find out which members of the medical team are covered by your insurance. For instance, you may need to follow up with your insurance company if the surgeon you have decided on will be bringing in a specialist to assist. While your surgeon may be in network, that doesn't mean everyone in the operating room is. Depending on who your surgeon uses, that specialist may or may not be covered by your insurance: if they are not covered, you will be paying their bill out of pocket. If your policy does cover bariatric surgery, you may be asked to show evidence that you medically qualify for the surgery before your claim can be approved. Evidence your insurance company may ask for includes:

- Having a BMI of 40 or greater.
- Having a BMI of 35 or greater, along with a weight-related health issue. (e.g., type 2 diabetes, high blood pressure, sleep apnea)
- Proof that you have tried and failed at weight loss through more traditional methods of diet and exercise.

In addition, you could be asked to complete a few extra procedures not required by your surgeon before your insurance will cover the surgery costs. Being able to cover every requirement for all insurance companies is beyond the scope of this book, but here are some of the more common insurance company requirements:

- Completed and documented medically supervised weight-loss program for up to six months.
- A psychological exam to ensure you can adequately address the changes associated with weight-loss surgery.
- Cessation of all tobacco and cannabis use before surgery.
- No evidence of substance abuse.
- A diagnosis of obesity or morbid obesity for a number of months or years.

If there is any chance that you have any of the following conditions, your doctor may require you to be tested or receive clearance from specialists prior to your surgery. You should ask your insurance company if these tests would be covered in addition to the surgery.

- Sleep apnea.
- Cardiovascular disease.
- Kidney or liver disease.
- Digestive disorders, such as Crohn's disease.

Even if you fit all your insurer's requirements, there's a chance you will be denied due to underlying health issues that make the surgery too complicated to perform. If you have one or more of the following conditions, the chances are high that you will not be approved for surgery:

- Severe blood clot issues.

- Any type of heart, neurological, or other conditions that make safe use of anesthesia impossible.

There is also the chance that your surgery could be canceled after you've been wheeled into the surgery room. If you have had past surgical work in or around your stomach and intestines, there is a chance that significant scar tissue has built up. If this scar tissue is too abundant or makes your procedure too difficult or dangerous for your surgeon to complete, they may cancel the procedure at the time of surgery.

Medicare coverage

When it comes to Medicare coverage, the good news is there are few differences in qualification you need to show for bariatric surgery. Medicare covers all three major forms of surgery (duodenal switch, gastric band, and gastric sleeve).

Finding the Right Surgeon

Finding the right surgeon is one of the most important parts of your entire weight-loss journey. It can mean the difference between a smooth recovery and a weight-loss journey filled with complications. Nothing is perfect, though, and even after a thorough vetting, you could still end up with complications and long-term issues with your tool. But taking the time to do your due diligence will reduce these chances significantly.

Start with referrals

Talk to your insurance company to find out if there are surgeons that are in network for your plan. Ask your primary care doctor for recommendations; perhaps they've had other patients who have had the surgery. If you have friends, family, or coworkers who have gone through bariatric surgery, ask them about it—they should have some good input. Even if the surgeon they used is not local, their stories can help clarify some things for you or reveal considerations you haven't thought of.

Try social media

If you don't know anyone who has gone through this surgery or you would rather not let many people know about your decision, join a few social media groups associated with bariatric surgery. Look for groups based around support and recovery; they should have lots of useful information. Also look for groups that are local to where you are planning on having your surgery. This is a good way to get reviews of doctors you are considering. Additionally, these local groups can give you an opportunity to increase your support team and maybe even find a workout/support buddy postsurgery.

Check credentials

Once you have a few doctors' names, investigate their certifications. If you are in the United States, the doctor should hold a certification with the American Society for Metabolic and Bariatric Surgery (ASMBS). You can get a list of ASMBS-qualified doctors from their website (https://asmbs.org/patients/find-a-provider). Also investigate the hospital where your surgery is going to take place. Is the hospital accredited with ASMBS's Metabolic and Bariatric Surgery Accreditation and Quality Improvement Program? Since this accreditation demands very high standards for a bariatric surgery program, it should be fairly easy to find this information. The simplest way to investigate if your chosen hospital holds this accreditation is to check their website. If it doesn't, see if there is another one that does. And this brings up another important point: Is the hospital's location convenient? You'll have to make a few visits before and after your surgery. Of course, with the increase in telehealth, this may not be as much of an issue—but ask about that, too.

Conduct interviews

Once you've narrowed your list to two or three top surgeons, set up appointments to talk with them. Remember, you are hiring a specialist, so you should be going into this meeting with questions to ask them. Check with the surgeons' offices to see if they offer informational sessions, as these can be good opportunities to hear not only from the surgeon and his or her staff but also from some of their past patients. If they offer any type of support group or classes, take the time to attend one or two of these. It's another good way to meet other patients, to hear any issues they may be having with their weight loss—whether associated with their surgery or with old habits creeping back in—and to possibly increase your support network.

By the end of your research into finding a surgeon, you should know all of the following about your surgeon and their surgery program:

- The number of surgeries they performed in the last year.
- Their qualifications and certifications.
- Your comfort level when talking about personal issues concerning your obesity.
- How satisfied other patients are with the surgeon.
- What post-op support they offer.

- What they recommend as the right procedure for you, and their reasons for recommending it .
- Their success and failure rate for the procedure they suggested for you.
- What other specialists will be assisting in the operation, as it can be a surprise expense with both self-pay and insurance.
- How their office deals with all insurance matters around your surgery.
- What you will be required to do before your surgery.
- If the surgeon is in your insurance network.
- How much self-pay will cost. (if you will not be using insurance)
- How long your recovery will be: how long it will be until you can go back to work and resume other normal activities.

If you don't have insurance and can't afford the out-of-pocket expenses, there is one more option: to go international.

Medical Tourism: Bariatric Surgery in a Different Country

More and more people are going to foreign countries for bariatric surgery. For many people, this choice is based primarily on budgetary concerns. While surgery can be less expensive in a different country, if you do go abroad, it's even more important for you to do your due diligence than when you have the surgery locally. The suggestions for finding a surgeon in the previous section apply here as well. One big limitation can be getting to speak with your surgeon before your procedure. This could be more difficult for a few reasons: language barriers, time zone differences, and cultural considerations are a few. If this is the case, you will have to rely more on patient reviews. The surgeon's office should be able to give you a few names to work from but look on your own. Social media is a good place to start.

There is no universal standard of care when it comes to bariatric surgery. But there are a few accreditation boards that do a good job of vetting bariatric programs around the world. The Joint Commission International (JCI), International Society for Quality in Health Care (ISQua), and the Surgical Review Committee (SRC) all have procedures to accredit different medical facilities. Though not perfect and though there can be differing standards for each organization, these are good places to find more information and increase your chances of a successful surgery.

There are a few additional risks that come with international bariatric surgery. Pre-op work and post-op follow-ups can be more difficult, especially with long-term care. Without good surgical documentation, some physicians in your home country will not take on patients who have had surgery abroad due to liability for future complications. Long-distance trips can increase the chances for clotting issues like deep vein thrombosis and pulmonary embolisms because you won't be able to move around as much as you need to. Also, any infectious disease or lack of immunity toward pathogens local to the area can increase the risk of complications.

There is much more to investigate if you want to have your bariatric surgery performed internationally, and those considerations are beyond the scope of this book. But if you're considering this option, I've listed some sources below where you can start your research. I can't advocate for or verify the validity of these organizations, so please do your due diligence, and evaluate multiple sources of information to ensure you find the right doctor and medical facility.

- Surgical Review Corporation: www.surgicalreview.org
- American Society for Metabolic and Bariatric Surgery: asmbs.org/patients/medical-tourism
- International Federation for the Surgery of Obesity and Metabolic Disorders: www.ifso.com
- Joint Commission International: www.jointcommissioninternational.org
- MedicalTourism.com: www.medicaltourism.com

Chapter Summary

Finding the right surgeon, knowing what procedure you are going to have, and lining up how this will all be paid for is the foundation of everything else to come. The time you put in will significantly improve your chances with your weight loss and improved health.

Yet before going on to all the things you need to do to prepare for this surgery, it's important to first understand the two main foundations of your success. These foundations are significant to every part of this journey to such a degree that without them, you will fail. The first foundation is the three pillars of weight loss and health. These pillars are not exclusive to bariatric surgery but to anyone who is trying to lose weight and become healthier. You must have all three in your plan if you want to be successful. The second foundation is the rules of the tool. As mentioned before, this procedure is a tool to help you lose weight and become healthier. These are the rules you need to follow to use this tool effectively.

36

SECTION 2: The Foundations of Your Success

Chapter 3: The Three Pillars of Weight Loss and Health

When it comes to weight loss and building a healthy life, there are three basic things you *must* focus on to succeed:-

1. Your nutrition
2. Your exercise
3. Your mindset

Each of these pillars by themselves can help you lose some weight or prevent you from gaining more weight over a short time frame. But rarely does anyone want their weight loss to last for a few months; most people want to lose weight and never regain it. Yet losing weight and maintaining that weight loss without focusing on all three pillars is extremely difficult, if not impossible. Because of their importance, each chapter in the second half of this book has a section dedicated to each pillar. In this way you will be able to see how you can work on keeping this foundation solid.

Nutrition

We all know eating too much can make us fat, yet it's hard to figure out what the right amounts are. I would guess that most people don't have a clue about how to eat in order to lose weight. I wouldn't call that a failure: with hundreds of diets, each giving different and sometimes contradictory advice—eat five small meals a day, fast on alternate days, up your protein, eat like a caveman, drastically reduce fat consumption, never eat bread—it's almost impossible to know what is right. For many people this is why bariatric surgery is a great option: it removes much of the mystery and confusion about food consumption and provides you with a single set of guidelines to follow. After your weight-loss surgery, your diet and manner of eating will change, depending on where you are in the progression of your weight loss.

But although there will be restrictions on the amount of food you can eat due to the surgery, it's not foolproof. There are still ways to cheat the system, whether you intend to or not. Some of these cheats come from a simple lack of knowledge—too little education on the rules you need to follow (such as eating and drinking at the same time, grazing, not eating enough protein, and more that I'll explain later). Other times these cheats result from old eating and lifestyle habits and desires that reenter your life. It's these cheats that can make the eating and nutrition part of weight-loss surgery more difficult than you expect.

A client of mine who had gone through bariatric surgery stalled out on her weight loss after about eight months post-op. We started to look for changes in her life that could be contributing to this lack of weight loss. I had her keep a food journal for a few days. This was less about listing everything she ate than about increasing her awareness of what and when she was eating. It's not always bad food choices such as ice cream and chips that are to blame but often the quantity of food and why it's consumed. In this client's case, the food log showed that she was indeed eating more food than she should, mostly by grazing instead of eating distinct meals. Because she was grazing, or just eating a little bit here and there between meals, she created a situation where she never felt full. And this meant it was all too easy for her to add more food into her day. On top of that, her food journal also showed that her new job created new stresses, and she was eating more to cope with that. After a few months of working with a registered dietitian to help her reestablish a better meal schedule and food choices, she started to see a loss in weight again.

While bariatric surgery helps with limiting food, it isn't a cure for bad food choices and bad food habits. These habits and choices may go away for a while, but if you are not actively working to create good eating habits, they will come back and undermine your efforts.

Exercise

Many people think that exercise is key to losing weight. But the most effective tactic for weight loss is paying attention to nutrition; exercise is not a substitute for healthy eating habits. Even people who haven't had weight-loss surgery will only experience minor weight-loss effects from exercise—it's actually a poor substitute for weight loss.

Think about it in terms of numbers, specifically numbers of calories. If you ate 3,000-plus calories a day presurgery, and postsurgery your max limit is 1,200 calories, then you are going to lose weight thanks to that 1,800-calorie deficit. If you exercise, such as walking for sixty minutes, you'll burn about 300 calories. When you look at the daily difference between that 1,800-calorie deficit with weight-loss surgery compared with the 300-calorie deficit with exercise, you can see why exercise shouldn't be seen as a major part of your fat loss but more of an assist. But I'm not giving you an excuse to not exercise; instead, this is a lens that will help you see exercise in a different way.

So, exercise isn't a weight-loss star. But it does shine in almost every other aspect of a healthy life. It promotes lower blood pressure, helps you sleep better, bolsters your immune system, builds stronger and more fatigue-resistant muscles, gives you stronger bones, improves brain function, strengthens your heart and lungs, helps you move easier, lowers your A1C, reduces anxiety and depression, reduces the risk of cancer, improves digestion, and increases your self-esteem and energy level, among many other things.

I've personally seen how exercise has changed people's lives that had very little to do with losing body fat. These changes may not read as significant, but to my clients, they are huge positive steps. It's being able to lift the 50-pound dog food bag without asking for help, going on a walk with friends and keeping up easily, getting up and down off the floor without struggle, having the confidence in their bodies to do activities that were once thought of as impossible. While their exercise has some impact on their weight loss, the big payoff is how it improves their quality of life.

If you're not exercising regularly, you're leaving a lot of positive, healthy results by the wayside. Regular exercise may not be the magical key to weight loss, but it is part of the secret to overall health and well-being.

Mindset

Mindset is the pillar that ties everything together. While bad habits around diet and exercise can be part of the reason that you need this surgery in the first place, it's an unhealthy mindset that allowed these negative habits to grow. Everyone who undergoes this surgery shares some traits and behaviors, but what got you to the point of obesity is unique to you. While mindset is the pillar most people ignore, paying attention to your own unique issues and finding a healthy path to managing them is crucial to your success. This surgery provides you with a tool, a tool

41

that triggers the physical transformation of your body. But your mental transformation—how you think about yourself, how you cope with stressful situations, your attitudes toward food, and more—requires a different kind of tool, one that there's no surgical help for. That's a mindset adjustment. Just as you might learn a new way of cooking, you'll benefit from discovering a new way of thinking about yourself, your past, and your future. You may begin rethinking some ideas you've had about yourself in several areas. You may feel you're getting to know a whole new you.

How this tool changes your body will affect you as a person in different ways. Some people will look at you differently; some people will actually "see" you for the first time. You will hear comments that are meant to be nice but can come off as hurtful. Some people in your life may not like how you have changed, and they will disappear, or their behaviors and attitudes toward you may change—and unfortunately, not always for the better. This isn't an easy path. As with exercise and nutrition, getting a professional to help can go a long way. If you decide to go this route, take the time to find a mental health professional who truly supports you and your journey. You'll want someone you feel comfortable with but who still will challenge you. Although you will go through a psychological assessment before your surgery (which I describe in the mindset section of chapter 5), it is limited to one or two sessions, which is really not enough to create a change. To truly build a strong mindset around the changes this surgery brings, you need to be dedicated to putting in the time and effort to make the changes you need. I would suggest that if you don't already have a mental health professional, take time before your surgery to find one. It may take some effort, but you and your weight-loss success are worth it.

One of my clients had never talked with a therapist before her psychiatric evaluation that was part of her presurgery requirements. Around six months post-op her weight loss came to a halt, and she actually started gaining. She began to realize that maybe there is more to this journey than diet and exercise. I mentioned adding a therapist to her journey, yet she didn't really think that was necessary. When, after a few more months, she still wasn't seeing a weight loss, I mentioned therapy again, as a way to help her uncover what part of her mindset was keeping her from what she really wanted. At that point she was more open to the idea. Through a bit of trial and error, she found a therapist who fit her needs and personality. A few months after that, her weight loss started again. While I can't say for sure that the therapy is what did it, her work on her mindset did help her discover some habits and thought patterns that improved her self-awareness. She still feels she has a long way to go, but as she says, "Now that I see what I need to do, the journey is more exciting."

As Kelly McGonigal, PhD, writes in her book on the science of self-control, *The Willpower Instinct:* "Without self-awareness, the self-control system would be useless. You need to recognize when you're making a choice that requires willpower [such as a craving or want]; otherwise, the brain always defaults to what is easiest." Making the right choice in different situations—when you're at a party, feeling blue, or even celebrating something—requires more than willpower. You need to know why you're eating—hunger, boredom, anxiety? This approach requires you to know yourself and your motivations so you can make choices that are in line with your goals.

Taking time to understand yourself, your habits, and your strengths will only boost your success with your weight-loss journey. When it comes to being successful with your weight loss, getting these three pillars right is critical. There is a good chance one or more of these pillars is not really that strong in your life, and that is fine.

Awareness of the pillars and of your strengths and weaknesses is a good start. What you will see in this book, then, is a discussion of how you can prepare and proceed for success with all three pillars. And if you're anxious about how to handle nutrition, exercise, or changes in your outlook postsurgery, you'll find help with that, too.

Chapter 4: The Rules of the Tool

In addition to the three pillars of weight loss, there are eight rules called the rules of the tool that you will need to integrate into your daily life to get the most from this tool. The following eight rules give you a great starting point on using your tool the right way.

1. Drink water.
2. Don't eat and drink at the same time.
3. Get enough protein.
4. Limit the length of your meals.
5. Avoid slider foods.
6. Always measure the volume of your food.
7. Exercise.
8. Stay connected.

These rules are not something I created; they are guidelines that most every surgeon and dietitian in the bariatric field will recommend. They may have slight modifications around timing and protein quantity, but these rules are well established as the best way for you to lose your excess body fat. When you read through all these recommendations, you may find that there are a few rules that are the polar opposite of the habits you have now. Habits like not consistently drinking water or gulping it, being a fast eater, not exercising consistently, or grazing on snacks throughout the day. It's these little things that you may not even think about too much before your surgery that can get you in trouble once you have this tool. Pick your battles, though; as you read through these rules, you may find that there are a few that are more difficult to implement than others. If that is the case, focus on those first; you can come back to the others over time.

How can you start practicing these rules now?

Rule of the Tool 1: Drink Water

Rule of the Tool 2: Separate Drinking from Eating

While drinking water and not eating and drinking at the same time are different rules, they are so intertwined that it's impossible to talk about one without mentioning the other. But before I go into how to put these into practice, I want to spend some time talking about why you need to drink water. This may seem like a silly thing to discuss, but many people don't drink water or understand the implications of dehydration and how it can affect your weight loss.

The importance of drinking water

You will be asked to drink a minimum of 64 ounces of water daily once you get to the other side of your surgery. If you don't already have a strong habit of drinking water, then this needs to be a focus as you prepare. Even if you do already drink water, there will be some changes you probably will have to make. The habits I am talking about are *how* you drink water and *when* you drink water. While before your surgery this isn't an issue, it will become much more important after the procedure. How and when you drink water have probably flown below your radar most of your life, so changing these habits can be slow going. Because of this, I suggest that you start working on them at least six weeks before your surgery date. Yet before we talk about the how's and when's of drinking water, if you are someone who doesn't drink water constantly, we need to talk about *why* drinking water is important.

Water is by far the most vital nutrient that all living things need. Since we don't have the water-storing hump of a camel, getting enough water daily is critical to your health because it enables many necessary functions:

- Water is the prime delivery system for transporting nutrients and oxygen to the cells, including those in the brain.
- Water allows your muscles and joints to function properly.
- Water moves toxins and wastes out of the body.
- Water lets the body take in vitamins and minerals, along with many other necessary substances.
- Water helps regulate your body temperature.

If you don't drink much water during the day, recognizing the symptoms of dehydration can be difficult. For you, these symptoms are a normal state; if you feel uncomfortable or off, you don't attribute that sensation to a lack of water. But if you usually feel any of the following symptoms of dehydration, then you should look at your water-drinking habits:

- General thirst
- Lethargy or lack of energy
- Headaches
- General feeling of weakness
- Dark yellow urine

More severe dehydration symptoms include:

- Sunken eyes
- Very dry skin
- Rapid heart rate
- Fainting
- Very dark brownish urine

The consequences of dehydration

For most people, the symptoms of dehydration are enough to prompt them to drink some water. Our bodies are 60 percent water overall, so it makes sense that if you drink water infrequently, not only will you feel the symptoms of dehydration, but you can also set yourself up for some negative physiological complications. Being dehydrated can cause various health issues, including:

- **Reduced ability to concentrate and lower overall mood.** The brain is 75% water so even a 1 percent loss in hydration can cause "problems with cognitive performance . . . [that] include poor concentration, increased reaction time, and short-term memory problems, as well as moodiness and anxiety."[2]
- **High blood pressure.** Chronic dehydration can increase blood pressure: a lack of water in the cells prompts the pituitary gland to release a chemical called vasopressin. Vasopressin constricts blood vessels, and this increases blood pressure, leading to hypertension, which can lead to heart disease and stroke.
- **Shrinking joint cartilage.** Dehydration can cause the cartilage (which is up to 80 percent water) in your joints to rub together, eventually causing

48

weakening and wear over time. Over time, dehydration can cause cartilage to wear out completely; as it degrades, you'll experience long-term pain in the affected joint.

- **Muscle cramps.** Dehydration causes involuntary contractions of muscles. Anyone, not just athletes, who is minimally active and doesn't take in enough fluid can be prone to the involuntary muscle contractions we call muscle cramps.

- **Possible toxin buildup**. New, but limited, research studies shows that rapid weight loss can increase the amount of environmental toxins called persistent organic pollutants (POP) that build up in fat cells.[3,4] POP causes a variety of negative health effects, including cancer and immune system suppression. Adding extra water into your day may help your body remove these toxins. This area of study is still quite new, and there are still many unanswered questions around weight loss and toxin release. In any case, drinking water can only help.

The easiest way to avoid these complications is to add more water into your day. A typical adult needs approximately 64 ounces of water daily. If you are getting less than this, you don't need to jump directly to the 64 ounces. Start slowly, adding about 10 ounces a day more to whatever amount you drink now. You may find as you get closer to the goal amount, you will start to feel better and less fatigued. Of course, as you start to drink more water, you will have to go to the bathroom more often. You may find this frustrating, but it's worth the effort—think of it as a great natural way to take a break from whatever you are doing.

Water intake post-weight-loss surgery

Drinking sufficient water is as important for weight-loss
surgery patients as it is for anyone else. But there is a
difference in *how* you can consume your water. The
surgery reduces the stomach capacity of a bariatric patient
from 1 quart (32 ounces) of food and water to around 2
ounces. This makes consuming enough water more
challenging. In addition to the stomach-size limitations,
additional restrictions around drinking and eating can make
getting enough water even more difficult. This all makes a
focus on drinking water at very specific times and in very
specific amounts very important.

How to drink water after bariatric surgery

Presurgery *how* you drink isn't something you give much
thought to. But it becomes a big deal after your surgery.
With a smaller stomach capacity, if you are someone who
likes to gulp your water, it will take only once to not want
to do that again. For most people who drink in this way,
one of two things happen: they will either vomit the water,
or they will experience pain that comes with the pouch
being quickly overfilled. So practice sipping your water. If
you are a "gulper," it will feel unsatisfying at first, but it's
important that you establish this new habit. There are a few
tricks you can try.

You can use a straw, because it will reduce the
amount of water you can drink at once compared with
gulping. Be aware, though, that using straws for the first six
weeks after surgery is strongly discouraged because they
can pull air into your stomach, which can cause a lot of
pain. After you've healed, check with your surgeon or
dietitian to see if they will clear you to start using a straw.
You can also pour your water into a 3-ounce cup. That
way, even if you drink it all at once, the total amount will

still be limited and won't cause any issues. Or you can take small sips separated by a few seconds to help control the amount of water you take in.

When to drink water

When you drink water during your day is probably the most important and most difficult habit for anyone who has had weight-loss surgery. Before the surgery, you'd drink when you felt thirsty; timing was never an issue. But once you have this tool, knowing when to drink water becomes much more important. The rule you will need to follow is to stop drinking water ten to fifteen minutes before a meal and then start drinking no sooner than thirty minutes after the meal is over. This rule's purpose is to keep you from emptying your stomach too quickly during and after a meal. Liquid moves through your stomach more quickly than solid food and will push some of the food you have eaten into your intestines faster. This quick emptying of your stomach pouch can promote you to eat again sooner than you should, which is about every three hours. These excess meals can slow, or possibly stop, your weight loss. In addition, drinking water while you eat can decrease your stomach's sensitivity to being full. The section "Has your stomach stretched?" in chapter 9 goes into more detail about this. Technically, this careful timing of your water intake isn't necessary until some weeks after your surgery. But developing the habit before your surgery can be a big factor in the amount of weight you can and will lose. It's also a habit that needs to last forever, so practice it early for the most success.

So, what should this drinking habit look like? Here's a sample schedule that shows how you can drink 64 ounces of water each day—that's the minimum amount you need.

Eating and drinking chart

6:50 a.m.	Water
7:00–7:20 a.m.	Breakfast
8:00–9:50 a.m.	Water
10:00–10:20 a.m.	Snack
11:00 a.m.–12:50 p.m.	Water
1:00–1:20 p.m.	Lunch
2:00–3:50 p.m.	Water
4:00–4:20 p.m.	Snack
5:00–6:50 p.m.	Water
7:00–7:20 p.m.	Dinner
8:00–9:50 p.m.	Water
10:00 p.m.	Snack

Many people find this timing around drinking to be difficult since it goes against years of never having to think about it. Yet there are a few things you can do to help drink the water you need and prevent the desire to drink during mealtimes. One is to make sure to drink enough water between meals. By getting enough water in the few hours between meals, you will not feel as parched while you eat. If the habit of drinking isn't too strong for you, set an alarm to take a sip of water every fifteen minutes. If an alarm is too intrusive, there are products that use less intrusive methods, like water bottles that light up at designated intervals to remind you to drink. If not having anything to drink during your meals is really challenging, try eating hydrating foods, such as a few grapes or an orange slice, to add some moisture in your mouth. Some people end their meals with a teaspoon of plain yogurt to help clear their palate. If none of that will work for you or if you are already feeling full, then taking a few *small* sips of water can help.

More tips for drinking water

What if you don't drink much water in the first place? Many people just don't like the taste of water. Depending on the quality of the water where you live, that can be a big factor. But there are a few ways to change that flavor or make it easier to drink:

- Water filtration systems.
- Alkaline water.
- Water flavorings, such as MiO, lemon slices, cucumber slices, etc.
- Ice-cold water.
- Drinking a glass at a designated time of day. (e.g., first thing in the morning)
- Water cups with timers or measurement lines to remind you to drink.

If water just isn't your thing, there are some alternatives, which include sugar-free lemonade, clear protein drinks, herbal teas, and sugar-free popsicles. If the liquid is clear and decaffeinated, it can be counted toward your water intake. Note: In the very early postsurgery stage when you are struggling to get through a 12-ounce protein drink *and* trying to get water in, life is much easier because you can count the protein drink as water. But before you begin to rely heavily on water substitutes, especially protein drinks, discuss it with your surgeon.

Rule of the Tool 3: Get Enough Protein

Along with fat and carbohydrates, protein is a macronutrient that helps your body function optimally. If you've never thought about how much protein you're eating in a day or which foods contain larger amounts, now's the time to learn. Eating enough protein daily can be key to the success of your weight-loss journey.

Why is protein so important?

If you look at an optimal postsurgery diet, you'll see that the focus is on protein. In fact, it may look like a high-protein diet since that macronutrient will be the focus of many of your food choices. But that isn't the case. There are nine essential amino acids your body doesn't make that you need in order to stay healthy. Since this tool significantly limits the amount of food you can eat, if protein isn't your focus, then you are jeopardizing many important aspects of your health. Additionally, getting enough protein daily benefits your weight loss. While fat is the primary source of energy your body draws on after your surgery, it's not the only source. Your body will also take a small percent of its energy needs from your muscle mass (protein): basically, it will choose to keep some body fat, instead using muscle mass as an energy source. Eating enough daily protein can slow down this muscle mass loss, improving your ability to move easier and with less pain. Additionally, muscle is one of the biggest energy hogs in your body, so the more muscle you have, the higher your metabolism will be, which will help you lose more weight over time.

Protein also helps suppress your appetite. When your stomach senses a higher concentration of protein, it

54

moves food into your small intestines more slowly, which means it takes longer before you will want to eat again. Protein can also help with your sense of hunger by reducing the amount of ghrelin, the hunger hormone, circulating in your body while simultaneously increasing the amount of a hormone called peptide YY. This hormone binds with specific receptors in your brain, reducing the sensation of hunger. So when you've had enough protein in your day, you are less likely to snack or want to overeat from hunger.

Getting enough protein daily will also improve your healing after surgery. While the body is healing, it requires more of two nonessential amino acids, glutamine and arginine, to help build more collagen and promote cell production. Also keeping up with your protein can also help you reduce the amount of hair loss that comes from this surgery. Chapter 8 goes into more detail about hair loss and ways to control it.

Hopefully you can see why protein is pushed so hard with this tool and how it can benefit you in various ways. The next question is how much protein do you need to eat daily to take advantage of these benefits?

How much protein should you have in a day?

For the sleeve and gastric bypass surgeries, you should be shooting for a minimum of 65 grams of protein per day with the goal of getting 85 to 90 grams daily. For the duodenal switch, your protein levels are higher: a minimum of 80 grams with a goal of 95 to 100 grams each day. The amount of protein will be higher as you get further from your surgery and may increase more depending on your exercise program. This amount of protein can be daunting at the start since you are eating such small amounts of food. Given the limited space in your stomach for food and the importance of protein to your health, you should be focusing first on getting your protein. If, early on, you're

not getting your minimum grams of protein each day, talk
with a dietitian about some strategies you can use to get
more protein into your meals. They may suggest adding in
a protein shake or drink to help supplement your protein
needs. These protein drinks should be a temporary addition,
given that you will feel fuller and eat less when you focus
on your protein coming from more solid foods. If you are a
vegetarian or vegan, you might encounter some other
limitations, but plant-based protein supplements are more
widely available, so finding something that works for you
shouldn't be too difficult.

Quality complete protein

Finding the best sources of protein is important not only for
your overall health and success of the surgery but also for
convenience. Below is a partial list of high-quality proteins
that can help you achieve your protein goals.

High-Protein Meats (grams per 4 ounces)

Chicken breast	26
Ground turkey	23
Ground pork	22
Lean ground beef	21
Light canned tuna	17
Shrimp	12

High-Protein Plant-Based Foods (grams per 4 ounces)

Peanuts	17
Soybeans	14
Almonds	14
Pistachios	13
Cashews	10
Cooked navy beans	10

Black beans	8
Hummus	6
Green peas	3
Spinach	3
Avocado	3
Asparagus	3

High-Protein Dairy (grams per 4 ounces)

Cheddar cheese	25
2% cottage cheese	12
Low-fat Greek yogurt	12
2% milk	4

As a reminder: some high-protein foods, such as nuts and cheeses, are also high in fat. While eating large portions of these foods will help you get your protein grams for the day, you may be exceeding your calorie needs due to the high fat content. And if you've had the gastric bypass or duodenal switch, excess fat in your diet can lead to bowel movement issues due to the lack of fat absorption that these procedures offer. To avoid these extra fat calories, choose cheeses and nuts as snack foods or in combination with lower-fat choices. Eating too much protein in a day has its downsides as well. Eating a large quantity of protein increases your risk of cancer,[5, 6, 7] constipation, and kidney damage for people with preexisting kidney issues. While you need to eat a large quantity of protein for these risks to show up, it is still good to be aware of some of these risks. Yet a more common issue is not eating enough protein, and if you are experiencing one or more of the following symptoms, you may need to up your daily protein intake:

- Fatigue
- Depression

- Muscle mass loss and weakness
- Slower recovery from sickness or injury
- Increased craving for sweet and unhealthy foods
- Oversleeping or sleeping more than normal

You might make it a habit to "check in" with yourself throughout the day to see how you feel and reflect on your protein intake. For a lot of bariatric surgery patients, fatigue is one of the most common symptoms of low protein.

Try to spread your protein intake over the day

Avoid getting all your protein at the beginning of your day. While this doesn't matter to your body that much, it will affect how you eat throughout the rest of the day. Loading all your protein into the first few meals of the day can open up the rest of the day's menus to more carbohydrates and fats. A main protein at each meal will also make you feel more satisfied with your meal, which will reduce your desire to eat more often than you should.

Rule of the Tool 4: Limit the Length of Your Meals

This tool's main purpose is to limit the amount of food you can eat in one sitting. It's through this limitation that you will lose weight. Yet as effective as this tool is at limiting food intake, you can still cheat the system. Cheating, or bypassing the tool's main purpose, isn't something you'll be doing consciously or with purpose but instead comes from habits you've developed over the years. One way you can inadvertently add more food and calories to your day is by *not* having a distinct mealtime. This opens up the opportunity to eat more than you intend by eating small bites of food over the course of hours. With this way of eating, you never genuinely feel full, so you never have a signal to stop eating. When you give yourself a time limit for each meal, around twenty minutes, and pay attention to how you feel by the end, you shouldn't need or want to eat for a few hours. One of the most effective ways to do this is by slowing your eating through deliberate chewing.

Chewing your food more

The main purpose of the stomach is to break down foods to a point where the intestines can absorb the nutrients into the rest of the body. The way this is done is to transform the food into a paste-like substance. By chewing your food more and allowing the enzymes in your saliva to start breaking down the carbohydrates and fats, you are making it easier for your stomach to complete this breakdown more fully. This in turn increases the amount of nutrients that will be more easily absorbed in the small intestines. And with your smaller stomach, the digestion process can be more taxing. So, the more you chew your food, the less work your smaller stomach has to do.

Taking more time to chew each bite can also keep you from overeating. There is a point during digestion when your stomach will signal your brain that it's full. This "full" signal is typically on a twenty-minute delay. By taking the time to chew your food more, you will be keeping pace with this signal so by the end of your meal, you should start to feel the full signal kicking in.

Taking time to chew more adds a level of food enjoyment to your eating. This can be an important psychological addition to your meals. By eating slower and letting the food stay a little longer on your tongue, your enjoyment of that food can last longer. If eating slowly is something new to you, you should add this habit to your routine. Just like breaking the habit of gulping your water, slowing your eating will be beneficial to your overall weight loss.

Rule of the Tool 5: Avoid Slider Foods

A slider food is any food that moves quickly through your pouch or that will be quickly absorbed into your bloodstream. Broths, smoothies, yogurt, or any other heavy liquid foods would be considered slider foods for how fast they move through your pouch. Heavily processed, high-sugar foods are also considered slider foods because of how easily the sugar is absorbed into your bloodstream. It's the quick absorption that greatly increases your chances of experiencing dumping. Dumping is the term used to describe how your body reacts to a spike of sugar in your bloodstream. Chapter 7 goes into more detail about dumping. For now, just know it's something you want to avoid. Even if dumping isn't something you need to worry about too much (which is the case for the gastric sleeve), adding in these highly processed foods will spike your insulin levels and promote an increase in fat storage.

Some common slider foods are:

- Chips
- Crackers
- Pastries
- Sodas
- Veggie straws
- Pretzels
- Candy
- Chewable sweets
- Broths

- Smoothies
- Yogurt

For the first few weeks after surgery, it's impossible to avoid some slider foods like broths and yogurts. Your stomach is very tender, and liquid is all you should be eating at this stage. It's only after you have fully healed and are cleared to a full menu of food that you should start avoiding slider foods—though the highly processed, high-sugar foods and drinks should be avoided from day one.

How to avoid these types of food is straightforward. The easiest way is to just stop buying them. Not having them in your home significantly reduces your chances of eating them. In addition, start replacing these slider foods with healthier alternatives. Having access to healthy, high-protein snacks like nuts, eggs, cold meat, and shredded chicken will help to overcome hunger and cravings for sugary snacks. With yogurts, choose ones that have low or no sugar and high protein. It's this high protein that can signal the stomach to slow the movement into the intestines. Instead of broths, choose heartier soups like stews and chilis, which will leave you feeling full longer.

Rule of the Tool 6: Always Measure the Volume of Your Food

In the early days of working with bariatric surgery patients, I had a conversation with someone who had lost over 100 pounds from the gastric sleeve and had kept it off for more than three years. I was impressed when she said she had experienced very little weight gain that many people experience a few years out. I had to ask what her secret was. Her answer was quite simple: she just kept a close track of the volume of food she ate. She never allowed herself to guess at her portion size. By keeping her food volume in check, she dramatically slowed the time it took for her stomach to accommodate to more food. In other words, she maintained feeling full on less food for many months longer than her friend who had gone through the surgery at the same time. And this food constraint, she believes, was a big part of her success in losing the weight she needed to lose and keeping it off.

I have seen this same weight-loss success in a few of my own clients. They are very diligent in measuring their food volume with each meal, never allowing their eyes to tell them what four ounces of chicken is; they always measure it out. They are the first to admit it's tedious, but their dedication to building this habit made all the difference in their overall weight loss. I bring these stories up because one of the sneaky things that can happen after bariatric surgery is an increase in the amount of food you consume. The amount starts small—it has to, because there isn't much room. But after a while there is a gradual increase in the amount you can eat. One reason for this comes from guessing or overestimating the volume of food you are eating. At first you may be close to accurate, but with time what you may think is 4 ounces could in reality be 5 or 6 ounces. Over time that extra amount of food will add up. By measuring the volume of food for every meal every day, you can guarantee that you're eating the right amount of food. Additionally, when you are consistent with the volume of your meals, you will maintain a more limited capacity of your stomach. It's when people stop measuring the volume of their food that they notice they are able to eat more in one sitting. This brings on a fear that they have "stretched their stomach." In reality, it may be more of a sensory issue than a physical change in capacity. I go into more detail about this in chapter 9.

Additionally, the more often you practice this rule, the better you will be at estimating the volume of food when you are in situations where you can't measure your food, like eating at a restaurant or a friend's house. You may have noticed that I've focused on the volume of food and not the weight. This is because you need to know how much space your meal is going to take up in your pouch. While the volume and weight of some foods will stay consistent before and after cooking, the difference between the weight and volume of other foods can change significantly after cooking. This increase in the size of your meal will add more pressure to your stomach. Over time, your stomach will learn to accommodate this extra volume and give you the feeling that you have "stretched your stomach."

The more you practice this rule, the better your chances of maintaining a smaller portion size. Yet if this rule feels too daunting for you to do daily, then measuring your meals every few weeks can help "calibrate your eyes" to what different volumes of food look like.

Rule of the Tool 7: Exercise

You can't be successful in this journey without consistent, progressive exercise in your life. That means having a detailed plan that continues to challenge you in different ways. What that looks like is a significant focus of this book, so I will not go into much detail here. But just know that if exercise isn't part of your life now, it will need to be.

Rule of the Tool 8: Stay Connected

Your support team

Having a team of people to support you on this journey goes a long way toward your overall success. Depending on your social circles, this can also be a difficult part of your preparation, but there are ways to get what you need.

Following are a few examples that span the range from significant support to near none.

One of my clients, John, showed great success in his weight loss after his gastric bypass. A large part of this success came from his wife, who did everything she could to help him lose weight. She was at every appointment, meeting, and class. She took copious notes about everything that needed to be done and had John strictly follow the rules of the tool. She scheduled when he would eat (every three hours). She would have his water set up, plan all his meals, and calculate the volumes of food he ate. He told me on a few occasions that she was the only reason he was losing weight. I don't truly believe that was the case: John was also very dedicated to his weight loss. But I'm sure he would agree with me that his one-person support team gave him the foundation to lose 200 pounds. While it would be great if everyone could have a partner as supportive as John's wife, it's not in the cards for most people. You might find that you need to manage expectations for the people around you, and that you'll need to make sure they understand the changes that come from this procedure. Often families just don't fall into place with all the new systems around eating and exercise plans. You will have to help them help you. Amanda's case serves as a good example.

Amanda was a client of mine with a busy job, a husband, and two young children, so the time she had to dedicate to her weight-loss efforts was limited. At first, her family was somewhat resistant to making the changes she needed. That is, she discovered that her support team—her husband and kids—needed to be managed. They did want to help her, but they also resisted change. For Amanda to succeed, things like schedules, meals, and old eating habits needed to change for everyone, not just for her. In order to squeeze workouts into her schedule, she needed her husband to shoulder some of the errands she had been doing. This took some negotiations with him and adapting schedules to make it work. She told me it wasn't easy, and there were times when the workouts didn't happen due to schedules not aligning as planned. In addition, Amanda's meals were different from those of her family. She still ate meals with them, but most of the time her food was different from the family's. This bothered her. One form of support she needed was to feel as if she were eating the same as her family. This became easier for her when she realized what she wanted and passed the information along to her family. Their support was to make the meal feel more inclusive by eating the same foods Amanda ate, and not to make a big fuss around the small amount of food she was eating. This didn't all fall into place right away; in fact, there were many setbacks as the entire family adjusted to the new reality. But she knew her family was on her side, and by keeping communication open, she found a way to have her family support her needs.

And sometimes, there are people who face a near-total lack of support. That was Linda's situation. When we met, Linda told me that everyone in her circle was against her decision to have bariatric surgery and gave her all kinds of nonsensical reasons why she shouldn't go through with it. I give Linda a lot of credit: it's difficult to have everyone in your life tell you your decision is wrong yet still go ahead with it. When it came to finding support from others postsurgery, Linda developed a strategy to build a support system from people outside her immediate, unsupportive friends and family. She hired me to help her with exercise and to keep her on track with things like the rules of the tool and habit changes. She attended a few support groups, either in person or through social media. Some worked for her, and she dropped the ones that didn't. Over time, she found a few other women who lived near her home, and they would meet up for a walk once a week during which they would help each other with menus and just general venting and support. For Linda, finding support came slowly, and there were many pitfalls along the way. Her weight loss was a little slower than she wanted in part due to this lack of family support. Yet once she found a stable group of support people, she was able to renew her focus on her weight loss and stick with it.

These are just a few examples of how others who have undergone weight-loss surgery had support, some built in and some created from nothing. Yet they all knew it was important to their weight loss. So don't take this part of your preparation lightly, and be prepared to ask for or find what you need.

Roles to fill within your support team

When you are looking to build your support team, here are some of the roles that need to be filled:

- Mental health coach or therapist
- Personal trainer or fitness buddy
- Registered dietitian
- Postsurgery aide
- Support group of weight loss surgery peers
- A good friend

While you'll likely always want the support of a good friend, not all of these roles will be permanent fixtures in your life—a few, like a registered dietitian, might be around just long enough to get you oriented. But each person can contribute to your success.

Mental health coach or therapist.

If you are not aware of the triggers or weaknesses that contributed to your obesity in the first place, you can't expect this journey to be successful. In addition, the changes that come from losing so much weight so quickly can affect how you see yourself as well as how others react to your changes. Having a professional to help you navigate these changes in your life and your relationship with food will give you the mental and emotional tools to continue your positive changes. Be patient with finding the right person to take on this role for you. While they don't have to understand the ins and outs of bariatric surgery, they should be open to your decision. You should feel comfortable with this person and be willing to discuss sensitive issues with them. And you should be willing to do the work on your side to help change unhealthy habits.

One place to start is to request a list of therapists from your insurance company; this could help offset some of the expense. You can also ask your surgeon or a close friend or family member to recommend someone.

In addition, if you are feeling a bit overwhelmed with how to integrate all of this into your life, look into hiring a mindset coach. Note: mindset coaches are not a substitute for therapy. A coach is someone who can help you recognize bad habits and behaviors you have now and give you tools to change them. A therapist is someone who can help you uncover the reasons why you behave the way you do.

Personal trainer or fitness buddy

I've mentioned before that you need exercise for this surgery to be successful. If this sounds daunting or confusing, hiring a professional trainer is a good start. It might seem expensive but think of the cost as an investment in setting yourself up for success. You likely won't need a trainer long-term, but a few months to a year of guidance will give you the dedication, technique, and knowledge you need to develop a safe, smart fitness plan.

And if you have any movement limitations, hiring a professional will help you learn how to exercise safely and within your physical limits. A personal trainer can also act as a springboard to build your confidence to try new activities. The section "Start trying new things" in chapter 9 goes into more detail with this. If you don't already have a personal trainer and are considering one, the bonus section goes into more detail about how you can find one that will work best for you.

If you can't or don't want to hire a personal trainer, find a friend or two that you can work out with. As a matter of fact, even if you hire a personal trainer, you should look for a fitness buddy. Working out with someone else can be quite motivating: just having someone who is counting on you to show up pushes you to get up and go do the workout. Being with someone whose company you enjoy while you work out makes the sessions go faster, and if you don't like exercise, it can make the sessions less miserable. You can also combine these ideas and talk with a personal trainer about training you and your friend. This way you can get the best of both worlds, and your training sessions may be a bit less pricey.

Registered dietitian

Fundamental to this weight-loss journey is eating the right foods and following the rules around eating and drinking. If a registered dietitian is part of your surgeon's practice, you already have this support. Take advantage of the knowledge and experience these professionals offer. And if your surgeon doesn't offer these services, you can hire a registered dietitian to help you develop menus and eating plans and give you some advice around eating issues.

Postsurgery aide

When your surgery date rolls around, have someone with you who can help you take on some of the little tasks that will pop up. This help can make the day less stressful.

- You will need someone to drive you to the hospital and check you in.
- Someone can be nearby for a few hours after you come out of surgery to assist you before your first night's stay.
- Someone else can be on call to bring things to you or retrieve items you may have left at home.
- And, of course, have a driver take you home.

Of course, all of these roles can easily be the same person.

Support group of weight-loss surgery peers

Meeting regularly with a group of people who share a similar journey provides many benefits. You'll be able to talk over issues or concerns; they can help you make better choices and find answers to questions; and you can just meet new people who provide new perspectives. There are many different support groups out there. Don't take this part of your support team lightly; a review of different research studies shows that people who attended support group meetings have a positive association between that attendance and their weight loss.[8]

- One study reported a decrease in BMI of 42 percent for people with support versus 32% for no support groups.[9]

- One study reported an excess weight loss of 55.5 percent in support versus 47.1 percent in non–support groups.[10]
- One study reported an average BMI point decrease of 9.7 in support versus 8.1 in non–support groups within the first year after surgery.[11]
- One study demonstrated a correlation between the number of group meetings attended and the variance in weight loss within the first year.[12]
- Another study concluded that "patients attending psychotherapeutic interventions or support groups in combination with bariatric surgery appeared to experience greater weight loss results than patients treated with bariatric surgery only."[13]

Ask your surgical team if they offer or know of support groups you can join, or if they have other patients who are looking for a support buddy. Search on social media platforms for others who are going through the same thing (use search terms such as "bariatric," "gastric bypass," "gastric sleeve," or "weight loss surgery"). This may be a second-tier support level, but if you are having difficulty finding someone to be a part of your journey directly, this is a good choice. Even if you are hesitant to dive right in with a support group, simply joining one can be useful. Just by listening you'll learn a few tips and tricks and feel like you're part of a community, both of which can improve your chances of success.

A good friend

Of all the support members in your team, including professionals, it's those one or two good friends who listen to you unload your frustrations or laugh with you that are by far the most important. Having someone in your life to whom you can offload some of your daily commitments in order to free your own time for weight loss and health activities is massive.

Chapter Summary

This can seem like a big list of habits to work on and change, but don't become discouraged. If you are weeks or months out from your surgery date, you have some time to start working on making these changes. You don't need to be proficient with all these rules before your surgery, but you should have a plan for how to implement all these into your postsurgery life. As I mentioned in the introduction to this section, you may find a few of these rules more difficult to change than others. If you are in the pre-op period when you are reading this, then starting now is great as you will have more grace around messing up, as will happen. Yet after your surgery, you'll need to truly adopt the changes to get the success you are looking for. It's this first year where these habits come into play; later in the book I talk about this as crossing the first starting line. Start the journey to your new life by practicing and integrating these new habits into your life. You might even start a habit diary, noting the things that cause slip-ups and techniques for combating them.

Now that you have a good idea of what habits you need to work on to make using this tool a success to you, let's talk about what you will need to do to prepare for your surgery.

SECTION 3: Preparation

Chapter 5: Preparation for Your Surgery and Beyond

There will be many things you will need to do to prepare for your surgery. Some of this preparation will be focused on making your surgery as safe and painless as possible. Other parts of your preparation are more to set you up for an easier transition into this new life. This is the focus of this chapter. Chapter 6 will go into more detail on what your surgeon will ask of you and a general timeline on what you should be doing and when.

Using the Three Pillars to Help You Prepare for the Surgery and Beyond

Nutrition

Don't over prepare

Overpreparation is a trap many people get caught in during the run-up to their surgery. You are in this waiting phase of a few weeks to a few months before your surgery, and you want to feel prepared and ready to go. Yet too much preparation around the food you think you are going to eat after your surgery can be a waste of time and money.

It is surprisingly common how this surgery changes the taste of foods for many people. You may find that foods that were appealing presurgery are now unappealing. For example, a banana might taste too sweet or a potato might taste rancid. In a study about taste change and bariatric surgery, 73 percent of the participants reported significant change in the taste of foods. The most frequently reported change was in the taste of meat and sweet and salty flavors.[14] These were often reported as tasting substantially more intense than they did before surgery.

It's not just your taste buds that change. As the weight comes off after surgery, many people become more sensitive to smells. Because of the strong connection between smell and taste, food choices can be affected. It takes about six months after surgery for your olfactory sense to return to baseline (i.e., the level of someone who has never been obese).[15] You may notice after surgery that certain smells that didn't affect you much before the surgery start to become much stronger, and maybe even too strong for you to handle. Knowing that this may be the case, you may want to avoid cooking any strong-smelling foods for a while after surgery to avoid any ill effects that may come with those smells. It's for these reasons that many dietitians recommend that you don't stock up on protein drinks, powders, or bars before surgery. What tasted great before you went into the operating room may seem repulsive once you've gone home from the hospital. I know many of my clients end up donating or selling large amounts of protein drinks and powders due to their change in taste post-op. If you don't want to purchase a bunch of different protein drinks just to find out you don't like them, see if you can find someone who has gone through the surgery and found out the hard way that they no longer like the flavor of the food or drink they bought. There is a chance you can purchase just a few of these from them. The best place to find such a person can be through bariatric-friendly social media groups. Another good source would be your bariatric doctor's office, as some will take donations of protein drinks or powders from their patients who overbought only to have their tastes change.

Exercise

If you are someone who exercises consistently, continue with what you are doing. There's no need to increase your intensity unless that is part of your usual workout plan. If exercise isn't currently part of your life or if you feel overwhelmed, all you need to do at this stage is to just start a light exercise habit. The goal is to give yourself a chance to get used to frequent and purposeful movement. Just adding a few walks during the week is a good start. Once you are on the other side of your surgery and have been cleared for more strenuous workouts by your surgical team, then it's time to start really putting a plan together. This plan should consist of both strength training sessions and cardio sessions. If you're not familiar with how to put a workout program together, then consider hiring a coach or personal trainer to help you. The bonus section goes into much more detail around building a workout plan and how to find a personal trainer, questions to ask them, and estimated pricing.

Mindset

Most every surgeon will require a presurgery psychiatric evaluation to verify that you are truly focused on your success with this tool. While this requirement isn't directly tied to your safety during surgery, some people can get a bit tied up about it. So I want to take a bit more and explain this requirement further.

Presurgery psychiatric evaluation

For many people, weight can be tied to psychological considerations, and mental health issues can arise following surgery. The dramatic change that occurs with weight loss surgery can result in fear, anxiety, depression, and an increased risk of "transfer addiction," where a patient trades their addiction to food for an addiction to something else (such as substances, shopping, or gambling; see more in the mindset section of chapter 8). To ensure that a patient has realistic expectations about life after surgery, and that they are well equipped to handle the associated mental shift, most surgeons require clearance from a licensed psychologist. If your surgeon requires this, they may be able to provide you with a list of psychologists who specialize in weight-loss surgery evaluations. There are also practices that conduct online or telehealth visits for weight-loss surgery evaluations. Depending on the requirements of your surgeon, you may need to attend between one and three sessions. The visit itself will typically take sixty to ninety minutes. You will be asked to complete questionnaires before the appointment and to provide the psychologist with information about your psychological history, your past and current relationship with food, your support system, what you expect from weight-loss surgery, and how you think your life will change after surgery. The appointments tend to be casual conversations to explore more about you. After the appointments, the psychologist will provide a report to your surgeon with recommendation: either that you proceed with surgery, or that you address certain issues before moving forward.

While it's good to talk with a mental health professional before you go through this procedure, it is just an evaluation of your future success with your weight loss. Having a consistent appointment with a professional therapist to help you navigate these issues can help you stay on the path to long-term success. If you've never thought about talking with a therapist before, use the required psychiatric evaluations to get a feel for the experience. It may be a useful tool later in your weight-loss journey as you encounter changes in yourself.

Document the presurgery you

Many of my clients—or anyone who has gone through this surgery—say they regret not documenting the beginning of their journey. After a year or two, it can be difficult to remember your situation before the surgery or to realize how much you've changed. Having documentation of your presurgery self can give you a better sense of where you were and how much things have changed. If you are uncomfortable with how you look presurgery, you may find taking pictures of yourself difficult. If this is the case, ask a close friend or family member to take the picture—and not show it to you. Or just store the picture until sometime in the future when you feel more comfortable looking at your presurgery self again.

Some tips for taking your before and after pictures: When you take the photo, stand in a doorway or some other space that won't change, and wear the least amount of clothing you feel comfortable with. Both of these will help with the comparison as you assess your progress. In addition to the photos, measure your body. Specifically, measure the circumference of your arms, legs, chest, and abdomen before surgery and then once a month after. Don't rely only on the scale. There will be times when you won't see a change on the scale, and you'll feel frustrated. It will feel like you're stalling, but that stall in weight loss may be a combination of fat loss with water or muscle mass gain. Having before and after measurements can help you better see your changes.

For extra credit, document how you move. Keep track of what you can and can't do in terms of movement before surgery. Write down how you feel walking up stairs or getting up from a chair. Knowing your baseline when it comes to what movements hurt and where the pain is can help you when you start your workouts after surgery. If you are planning on working with a professional trainer, giving them this information can help them better customize your program. Just as your photos give you a visual way to track your progress, a movement diary lets you see your physical progress.

An additional way you can document your change is with a DEXA scan or a bio-impedance scale, which will break down your scale weight into more basic components such as water, fat, and muscle; this will help you set a realistic goal for fat loss and give you a baseline for your starting muscle mass. These machines can be found at doctors' offices, physical therapists' offices, or sports performance gyms. They can be costly, but they do offer a good amount of useful information, especially if you're someone who likes data.

Food funeral: Is it a good idea?

A food funeral, or mourning the loss of certain foods from your diet, is something a lot of people do before their surgery. It might feel like a positive mindset act, like a ritual to say good-bye to your old food favorites. But it's probably not something you should do since it doesn't come from a positive place: A food funeral is based around fear that you will never eat the foods you like again. This fear may be based on a perception that the surgery is a punishment and this is your last night of freedom before going to jail. If that's how you're thinking, you need to adjust how you are looking at your postsurgery life. This surgery and its results are actually your path to a freer, healthier life—and you can still enjoy those foods after surgery. There are no food restrictions once you are through the six-to-eight-week recovery phase. There are, of course, some things that will be different about what and how you can eat. As mentioned before, your taste buds may change after surgery. Your favorite foods may no longer taste as good; your new stomach may not accept the food you eat and dump it out; and the amount of food you are able to eat will be much smaller. Yet no one is telling you you can't at least try any food. Although you are free to eat the foods you love after surgery, you shouldn't take that as license to eat as you did before surgery. But if you are doing all the things that are asked of you so you can lose the excess body fat, having an indulgence infrequently throughout the year isn't likely to derail your overall goals.

There are also practical reasons to avoid a food funeral. If your doctor has you on a diet to reduce a fatty liver, then binging or overeating some foods just before your surgery can impair that diet, and that can make your surgery more complicated for the surgeon. And there's always a chance that your surgery could be postponed. Many people at the beginning of 2020 saw their surgeries postponed indefinitely due to the COVID-19 pandemic. If you had been on your "last meal binge" or in a "it doesn't matter" stage and then learned your surgery would not happen for a few months or more, you'd have more work to do once you do get the surgery. Instead of waving a mournful good-bye to some foods, spend your energy starting the difficult job of changing your relationship with food. Instead of diving headfirst into bad eating decisions with a food funeral just before surgery, look for a professional who can help guide you to making better, healthier decisions around food choices that you actually like and can live with long-term. And prepare yourself for the unexpected: when your taste buds change, you may find it's not as hard as you expected to make better food choices.

Two of my clients had moments of disappointment postsurgery where they found they couldn't eat the one food they loved. One client loved Snickers bars and told me that presurgery, she would eat them a few times a week. Another loved pizza; it was her go-to meal at least once a week. A few months after surgery, each tried her favorite food. It did not go well. The Snickers lover ate only a few bites of her bar, then experienced her first bout of dumping syndrome. The pizza lover found that her pie no longer tasted right; she thinks it was the oil or the dough. Both confided in me that they were disappointed and a little depressed that they couldn't enjoy their favorite foods anymore. Yet they were actually quite happy about it as well. They knew that the weekly Snickers bars or pizza wasn't a good choice—and they would never trade their weight loss and new freedom from obesity just to go back to those foods. About six months after they told me their stories, I asked each of them again how they felt about the loss of their once favorite foods. My client who loved Snickers said she hadn't even thought about it since, and after I brought it up, she admitted that she had no desire to eat one. The first thing that came to her was the memory of dumping after eating the first bar and how awful she felt.

The client who loved pizza found a different and healthier way to eat it; she ate only the toppings and a small pinch of the crust. And even with this new way of eating pizza, she found that having it just a few times a year was more than enough for her. While I don't know if either of these clients had a food funeral, I use these two stories to highlight that the loss of a favorite food wasn't that devastating. In fact, given the changes surgery brought, both were happy with those formerly favorite foods being a less significant part of their overall food choices. This will happen to you, too. I say it again and again: this surgery is the start of a new life with new habits and new choices. Don't fear it or mourn the loss of things that are not worth your time to mourn over. Instead, take the time to build the path where you want to go.

Chapter 6: What Your Surgeon Will Require for Your Surgery

There are many steps to get ready for your surgery; some will feel like little more than jumping through bureaucratic hoops, but others are crucial to the success of your surgery and everything that comes after. The following are some of the more common tests that you will be asked to take. Depending on your individual needs, your surgeon may have some more specific requirements for you. The main reason for these tests and requirements is to ensure your safety during and directly after your surgery. Following through with these requirements is one reason that this surgery is so safe.

Medical Tests You Will Need to Take before Your Surgery

Since this part of your surgery preparation should be extensively covered by your surgical team, I've listed a few of the more common tests along with a brief explanation for each one so you can better understand what will be asked of you.

If you have a history of heart disease, you will be asked to have an exercise and EKG stress test. The purpose is to test the overall function of your heart and possibly expose any issues that may make your surgery more dangerous. If you have any acid reflux or suspected abnormalities in your upper gastrointestinal tract, you probably will be required to take a barium swallow. This test consists of drinking a contrast so your surgeon can visualize what happens as you swallow. Having this information will reduce any surprises your surgeon may encounter. Gallstones are a common problem associated with rapid weight loss. There is a chance you will be asked to have an ultrasound around your abdomen to test for abnormalities or stones in your gallbladder. Since you will be sedated for this surgery, if you have any tendencies around abnormal stopping of breathing while you sleep, you may be asked to take a sleep study. The results from this study can help your surgical team know what to expect, and they will be better able to handle anything that comes up during your surgery.

You will be required to take a blood test to check your blood count, electrolyte levels, and kidney and liver function. You may also have a test of your iron level to see if you are deficient. As a note, you may test fine on your iron level pre-op but become deficient after surgery, so if you are experiencing any of the symptoms that come from a low iron count, you may want to get retested. The section on multivitamins in chapter 7 lists some of the more common symptoms that come from iron deficiency.

Four to Six Weeks before Your Surgery

Stop drinking caffeine

You will not be asked to stop consuming caffeine until after your surgery, but if you are someone that loves their coffee or tea, this can be a challenge to quit. Taking a few weeks before your surgery to step down your reliance on caffeine will help mitigate the withdrawal symptoms. So why is it that you shouldn't be drinking caffeine after your surgery?

Caffeine is a known diuretic. As mentioned before, drinking water is very important after surgery. If you are also drinking caffeinated drinks, then you are pulling water out of your system faster than you would be without caffeine.

Caffeine contributes to bone loss. That's because it blocks the absorption of calcium into the bloodstream. Bariatric surgery by itself has a negative effect on calcium levels in your body, so while the effect of this blocking is small, this additional reduction in calcium will add up.

Caffeine irritates the stomach. Caffeine is known to increase stomach acid.[16] Drinking caffeine early in your healing process can damage your already sensitive pouch.

Stop drinking alcohol

Drinking alcohol during the first six weeks after your surgery, when most of your healing occurs, will irritate your stomach and can complicate your healing. So if alcohol is something you use frequently, it's strongly advisable to start tapering off starting three to four weeks out from your surgery. Chapter 8 goes into more detail about how this tool affects your sensitivity to alcohol and the possibility of an addiction transfer.

Stop using nicotine

Besides all the other unhealthy aspects of nicotine use, nicotine increases risks with surgery. There is a higher rate of heart and lung issues that make anesthesia more dangerous and will increase your chances of a heart attack during surgery. Take this very seriously. You will be tested the day of your surgery, and if the results come back positive for nicotine, your surgery will be canceled.

Two Weeks before Your Surgery

Stop drinking carbonated beverages

For many people this can be a tough habit to break, but it is one you need to really focus on. Here are a few reasons you should stop drinking carbonated beverages.

Added sugar and sodium. If you are drinking any type of regular soda, you are consuming excess calories in the form of sugar. Sugar has no nutritional value, and those extra calories will jeopardize your weight loss. And if you drink diet soda, sugar-free soda, or just plain soda water, you may be surprised to know that these drinks all contain sodium. This extra salt helps with the overall flavor of the soda, but it can have a negative effect on your health.

Negative effect on ghrelin. Some recent research indicates that carbonated drinks (with or without sugar) have an increased effect on the hunger hormone ghrelin.[17] Given that this tool reduces ghrelin's effects, it's unknown how the results of this mostly animal-based study could affect future weight gain, but it is something to keep in mind as you reach for that bubbly liquid. It's also in these last two weeks you may be asked to start your liver-shrinking diet. With the possibility of carbonated drinks increasing your sense of hunger, limiting how much you drink during this time may help get you through this stage of your preparation with less difficulty.

Bubbles. The bubbles in carbonated drinks are gas, and putting it in your stomach can add extra pressure to the walls of your stomach. Those extra gas bubbles can produce more pain as they press on your stomach. This is most evident soon after your surgery, when your stomach is extra sensitive. Also, some surgeons recommend against carbonated beverages because they feel that the pressure from the gas can inhibit the stretch receptors in your stomach pouch. This can set you up to eat more food than you need. I talk about this more in chapter 9 under "Has your stomach stretched?"

Start Your Pre-op Diet

If you're obese, there's a high chance that you have nonalcoholic fatty liver disease. This is when an excess amount of fat builds up on the outside of your liver. The pre-op diet focuses on reducing this fat on the liver so the surgeon can more easily access your stomach during surgery.

If you've been diagnosed with nonalcoholic fatty liver disease, your surgeon may put you on a diet just before your surgery date to help reduce the amount of fat on your liver. It's worth your effort because it reduces the complexity of your surgery, which increases your chances of the surgery being successful and free of complications.

Below is an example of what a typical day looks like for this pre-op diet:

- Breakfast: high protein (>15 grams of protein); shake or meal replacement
- Lunch: high protein (>15 grams of protein); shake or replacement meal, small apple or pear
- Dinner: 3–6 ounces lean protein; 1 cup vegetables or a small salad with light dressing
- Snack: small apple, string cheese, 2 ounces deli meat or Greek yogurt
- Water: You will also need to drink approximately 64 ounces of water daily (which can include broth, herbal tea, and protein drinks) and take a daily multivitamin.

This is just an example of what you may expect; the diet your surgeon supplies for you will take your individual needs into account. If you are living with diabetes, talk with your primary care doctor or dietitian before starting this diet to avoid low blood sugar. You should be aiming to get between 60 and 80 grams of protein daily while on this diet. This is a fairly restrictive diet, so ask your surgeon about adding fiber and a calcium supplement to help offset any negative effects.

A Week before Your Surgery

There is a chance that a few days before your surgery, you will be asked to go in for a blood draw for a final test of your vitals, such as your kidney and liver function. If you are on any blood thinners or take aspirin daily, you will be asked to stop those medications a week or so before surgery. This is also the time when you should fill any prescriptions you will need while you are in recovery. Having this medication with you will relieve you of that burden in those few days post-op when all you want to do is rest.

One to Two Days before Your Surgery

Packing and prep

Pack a few days in advance so you have time to make sure you have everything you'll want and need. While some procedures are outpatient, depending on your surgery and any possible complications, you should expect to be in the hospital for twenty-four to seventy-two hours. While it may be tempting to bring a lot of things to occupy your time, you're likely to find that you'll be sleeping, talking with nurses, or walking the halls (a post-op requirement!), so avoid the urge to bring a lot with you.

But there are things you probably need:

- Book or a tablet for reading
- Comfortable, loose-fitting clothing to wear home
- CPAP machine
- Glasses
- Hair bands
- Photo ID
- Insurance cards
- Lip balm
- Medications
- Mobile phone
- Portable battery bank or charging cables
- Mouthwash or sugar-free lozenges
- Slippers or slipper socks with a grippy bottom
- Sports bra
- Toiletries (deodorant, toothbrush, toothpaste, shampoo, hairbrush)

You may also wish to bring:

- Air freshener if you find you are sensitive to smells post-op (check if your hospital will allow)
- Ear plugs and/or sleep mask
- Heated blanket or heating pad
- Lotion

- Pajamas or loungewear (as an alternative to the hospital gown)
- Pillow (it's nice to have a small one that you can hug to your abdomen if you need to cough)
- Robe
- Shower shoes
- Small fan

The Day before and Surgery Day

The day before your surgery will probably be filled with anxiety and nerves, which is to be expected. Yet if you take a bit of time today to finalize some things for your surgery, you will feel much better.

First, make sure whoever is driving you to the hospital is still available and knows when you need to be at the hospital. Second, pack if you haven't already and double-check that you have all your important documents easily accessible for your check-in. And don't forget to enjoy your last drink of water before midnight. If your anxiety is high, you may want to distract yourself with a favorite movie or talk with a close friend.

In the next chapter, we look at the day of surgery and the first six weeks. This is a time that is filled with many new things like reintroducing food into your new stomach, dealing with buyer's remorse, and getting used to this new tool you now have.

SECTION 4: Your Surgery and the First Year

Chapter 7: Surgery and Your First Six Weeks

This is it: your surgery. After a period of thinking about it, planning for it, and maybe even talking about it, it's finally here. It may feel a bit scary, and you may find yourself second-guessing the decision in the days leading up to the surgery. (This may be especially true if you have had good weight loss on your pre-op diet.) Doubts are normal for this or any surgery. But remember, this surgery is a great opportunity to build a new life, an opportunity to be free of the confines of so much body fat and to experience the world differently. Of course, there may be difficult times ahead, but there will be nothing you can't overcome.

Here's a look at what's coming up in the six-week postsurgery phase. I've provided a look at your hospital stay with information about post-op pain and possible complications, an outline of your first days of eating and introducing solid foods and exercise, and a preview of what you can do to get started on your exercise plan.

The Hospital

Presurgery

The day of your surgery, your surgeon will want you to be at the hospital at least two hours before your procedure is scheduled, as the pre-op prep can take up to an hour and a half. During this time, you will have an IV started, and you will be given a blood thinner and leg compression sleeves. Your surgeon and anesthesiologist will visit you to have a quick chat about what to expect before they take you to the operating room. You can expect to be awake as they wheel your gurney to the operating room. You'll be given an oxygen mask as the anesthesiologist puts you under. The last part is now up to your surgeon and her or his team.

In-hospital recovery

Once your surgery is complete, you will be wheeled into the recovery room. Each surgeon has a different recovery schedule, and you can ask your surgeon what you can expect, but the following are likely to be a part of that process.

Get up and walk

One of the first things you'll be asked to do when you get to your room is to stand up and take a few steps. They aren't trying to be mean to you; just the opposite, in fact. Movement will help remove the gas from the surgery. If the surgery is done laparoscopically, then the surgeon will have filled your abdomen with some inert gas. The surgery team will remove most of it, but some will remain. Walking soon after surgery will help move the gas out of your body. Getting up and walking will also help prevent the formation of postsurgical blood clots. As an obese person, your chances of blood clots and pulmonary embolism (a blockage in an artery in your lung brought on by blood clots) are higher. The hospital will probably give you a pair of compression socks or use a leg compression massager to help reduce blood clots, but walking as soon as you can will greatly reduce your chance of clots. You will also be asked to walk at least three to five times a day while you are in the hospital, so even if you are not feeling too well, you should try to move as much as you can. This can include moving your arms and legs while you're in the bed or even some easy chair yoga.

Drink water

Your surgeon will want you to drink tiny sips of water soon after surgery. You may find this difficult. That's because your stomach is now much smaller, and also because your stomach will be very inflamed from the surgery. Consuming enough water after surgery is very important, and you will probably not be discharged until you are able to drink 1 ounce of water within a few minutes. The precise timing for that may be different for each surgeon, but the goal is to ensure you will be able to easily drink water once you are home.

I talked about practicing drinking water extensively in chapter 4 when discussing the rules of the tool, and now is the time to put that practice to work. For the first six weeks post-op, you should be sipping a few ounces of water every twenty to thirty minutes. This is the only time that eating (which you won't be doing much of at this point) and drinking at the same time is okay. That's because so soon after your surgery, it is difficult to get much of anything in your stomach before you feel full, so drinking water frequently will prevent dehydration. As the swelling goes down around your stomach, you will start to feel that you are able to drink 4 to 6 ounces of water more comfortably. It's about this time that you should start to practice the "no eating and drinking at the same time" rule. But don't rush this: staying hydrated at this point in your recovery is very important.

Possible Complications and Their Symptoms

Postsurgery pain

While most issues are a result of mild pain and discomfort, there are a few indicators that something serious is going on, and I want to put these symptoms right at the top. If you experience any of the following, contact your doctor immediately or call emergency services:

- A temperature higher than 100.5 degrees F / 38 degrees C.
- Difficulty breathing and/or chest pain.
- Redness and heat or severe swelling around incisions.
- Pus-like drainage around your incisions.
- Pain or swelling in your legs that isn't lessening or is increasing.
- Lack of any urination over twenty-four hours.
- Pain that is not relieved by your pain medication.

These are symptoms that don't occur too often, but it's good to be aware of them.

There are other pains after the surgery that are not as serious. Here's a look at some of the sources and how each can be alleviated.

Gas pain

Many patients complain of pain caused by the gas that is used during surgery. Your surgical team will attempt to remove as much of the gas as possible afterward, but they might not get it all. This gas isn't in your stomach but around your organs. After a few days, your body will absorb this gas, but in the meantime, you may feel some pain from the pressure of the remaining gas. Walking will help reduce the gas pain and will help the gas leave your body.

Incision pain

During the surgery, several incisions will be made around your abdomen for the surgical tools to access your stomach and intestines. For a few days to a week, you may feel some pain around these areas. This pain should be easily managed with the pain medication the hospital gives you. There may also be some bruising around the incision areas from the insertion and removal of different tools needed in the process.

There is a good chance that your surgeon will insert a drainage tube into your abdomen to help get some of the excess fluid out that comes from surgery. This drain, as it's called, will stay in you for a few days post-op, and it is not particularly comfortable. When they do finally take it out, many people describe the feeling to be downright weird.

Pain from swelling

The first few times you drink after your procedure, you might feel pain due to the swelling of the stomach lining. Due to this swelling, it will take very little water for your body to give you the "full" signal. The swelling will start to go down within a few days, making drinking less difficult. You may also feel pain from air getting into the new stomach. Again, with less space due to swelling, this air can add pressure to the stomach, making it uncomfortable. Walking around can help reduce this pressure fairly quickly.

Nausea and vomiting

Sometime soon after surgery, you may experience nausea. This could be triggered for a few reasons. This list is ordered by when you may experience these feelings, starting with soon after surgery to a few weeks to months later:

- Anesthesia or pain medication side effect.
- Not eating.
- Sensitivity to smells.
- Dehydration.
- Eating solid foods too soon after surgery.
- Not chewing your food enough.
- Eating past fullness.
- Drinking with a straw.
- Laying down soon after eating.
- Eating foods that are too dry, such as saltines.

While it is very rare, if you find that you can't keep anything down, you should contact your doctor. Vomiting can increase your chances of dehydration, so pay closer attention to your water intake if you have had a bout of vomiting. If your nausea is related to smells, apply a small amount of peppermint oil below your nose to help mask the odor. Also try to cook more bland-tasting food for a few days or get someone else to cook for you so you can avoid the kitchen aromas.

Possible Complications from the Surgery

As with any surgery, there is always the chance for complications due to the surgery itself or due to your body's response to the healing process. The most serious complications that come with this surgery have a very low chance of occurring, but again, knowing the signs will help you if they do happen.

If you have a competent surgeon, the likelihood of these complications becoming life-threatening are very low. If any of these complications worry you, make sure to bring it up with your surgeon before the procedure. It will help your peace of mind if you have a better understanding of what can be done to limit your risk of these complications. The following complications can show themselves very soon after the surgery:

Staple-line leakage

If the attachment point for the new pouch with the gastric bypass or the sealing of the stomach with a sleeve is not done properly, or a surgical staple pops out, fluid can leak, causing infection. While a staple-line leakage is a big risk of bariatric surgery, it's a well-understood issue, and there are very effective protocols in place to limit this from occurring. In fact, the rate of occurrence of a staple-line leak is very low (0.5 percent to 2 percent of patients). This doesn't mean a leakage can't occur later; it has less to do with the initial surgery than with how the healing takes place. Note: the risk of this is elevated for those who advance their diet before they are cleared to do so.
Usual signs of a leak:

- Fever (100.4 degrees F/ 38 C or higher)
- Trouble breathing
- Constantly high heart rate (120 bpm or higher)
- Increasing or not decreasing pain in the upper left abdomen

If you feel this is happening to you, you should contact your surgeon's office or call emergency services.

Unseen lacerations

There is a small chance that an errant cut around the stomach happens during the surgery and that your surgeon will miss it. This can lead to mild internal bleeding and possibly a slower recovery.

Adhesions

If you've had previous surgeries in and around the stomach, you could have adhesions. They form during healing, when tissues bind together. Depending on the severity of the adhesions, they could increase your overall surgery time since the surgeon will have to cut around all the tissue. In cases where the adhesions are significant, the surgeon could decide to not go through with the surgery because he or she can't get a good view of the stomach and intestines.

Complications in the First Few Weeks Post-op

Blood clots

Blood clots, also known as deep vein thrombosis, can be a very dangerous complication if left untreated. Because blood clots form when you're inactive, your hospital will have you up and walking as soon as possible. Even if you are not feeling great, try your best to get up and move around. If you keep moving, the chances of you developing a blood clot are quite small, less than 1 percent.
Usual signs of a blood clot:

- Redness
- Swelling
- Pain
- Loss of feeling
- Paleness in the area affected by the clot
- Inability to move the affected area

Gallstones

While this may not happen quickly after surgery, gallstones affect about 37 percent of weight-loss surgery patients.[18] The gallbladder is a holding area for bile, which breaks down fat. Created in the liver along with cholesterol, bile is transported to the gallbladder and held until it is needed for the breakdown of fat in the upper small intestine. Bile is usually able to keep the cholesterol particles suspended, but if cholesterol levels get too high, it starts to form stones in the gallbladder. Since this is such a common occurrence with bariatric surgery patients, most surgeons will put their patients on a medication to prevent the formation of gallstones.

Usual signs of gallstones:

- Sudden and rapidly intensifying pain in the upper right portion of your abdomen.
- Sudden and rapidly intensifying pain in the center of your abdomen, just below your breastbone.
- Back pain between your shoulder blades or the feeling of a "bear hug" around your middle.
- Pain in your right shoulder.
- Nausea or vomiting.

Hiatal hernia

Hiatal hernias occur when the upper portion of the stomach bulges through the diaphragm. There are different types of hiatal hernias, but the most common is a sliding hernia, a condition where the esophagus pulls the top part of the stomach above the diaphragm. While the gastric sleeve can increase the chances of a hiatal hernia, in many cases the surgery exposes this as a condition that existed before the surgery. This hernia can increase your chances of GERD, or gastroesophageal reflux disease, where the acid from the stomach is pressed up into the esophagus, creating a burning sensation after you eat or lie down. As mentioned previously, the gastric sleeve can increase the chance of this happening, while gastric bypass can reduce the chance. This isn't a very large issue, with about 4 percent of bariatric patients experiencing GERD or hiatal hernia after surgery.

Death

Death is by far the biggest fear with any surgery, including bariatric surgery. But your odds of survival are very, very high. The most recent data shows that this procedure has around a 0.13 percent chance of death within the first thirty days after surgery. That's around one out of one thousand patients. So while the population being operated on is in many ways very unhealthy due to obesity, the surgery that fixes the problem is quite safe. And of those who die within the first thirty days, not all of it can be attributed to the surgery. If the patient has been living with obesity for years or decades, there is a significant chance that this disease has taken its toll and the surgery happened too late.

Other Things to Look Out for during the First Few Weeks of Healing

Bowel movements

Given the limited amount of food you will be consuming, it's normal to not have a bowel movement every day at this stage of your healing. When you do, your stool will probably be on the softer side due to the smooth, liquid foods you've been limited to. If you go more than three days without a bowel movement, though, contact your doctor: it could be a sign of a bowel obstruction. If, on the other hand, you are having constant diarrhea or your stool is very wet, then you should call your doctor to talk about a treatment. If you let it continue, it could lead to dehydration, and you might wind up back in the hospital on an IV drip.

Dumping syndrome

If there's one most-feared side effect of bariatric surgery, it's dumping syndrome. While it can happen with any type of bariatric surgery, it's most common with gastric bypass patients. This is due to the loss of the pyloric sphincter, which controls how fast the digested food will move into the duodenum and small intestines. Dumping syndrome is caused when the stomach quickly "dumps" undigested food into your intestines. The most common cause of this comes from eating highly processed, sugary, fatty, or fried foods. There are two types of dumping: early dumping and late dumping. Early dumping is usually felt within ten to thirty minutes after eating. It's caused by the body trying to dilute the undigested food by moving water from the bloodstream into the upper small intestines. This increase in the amount of water in the small intestine brings on bloating, nausea, cramping, vomiting, and diarrhea. Additionally, this exchange of water from the bloodstream to the intestines can reduce your blood pressure, which increases your heart rate and can make you feel dizzy and lightheaded. Late dumping usually occurs one to three hours after eating. This occurs when the pancreas produces too much insulin in an attempt to deal with the high blood glucose levels from the high-sugar foods. This excess insulin then removes too much blood glucose, creating a condition known as hypoglycemia. When this occurs, you can feel lightheaded, shaky, sweaty, and weak and have a fast or irregular heart rate. Your chances of experiencing both early and late dumping syndrome increase significantly when you eat more highly processed or high-sugar foods like cake, doughnuts, and cookies.

How do you avoid dumping?

Dumping is directly related to eating high-sugar foods, aka slider foods. It can also be triggered by more sugary fruits, including bananas, mangos, and oranges. So the most direct way to avoid dumping syndrome is to avoid these types of foods altogether. Eating higher-fiber foods will slow down how quickly these sugars are absorbed into the bloodstream, which can keep you from experiencing dumping in the first place. Also eating more slowly, chewing your food more, and avoiding drinking during your meals will help.

Do you need medication for it?

You probably do not need medication for dumping. A small percentage of people have chronic dumping syndrome, and if that is the case for you, there are a few medications that can help with both early and late dumping syndrome. Talk with your doctor about what would work best for you. While dumping syndrome is unpleasant for most people, the symptoms typically wear off after a few hours or a day. But there's a silver lining: it's a great deterrent when in the future you reach for a candy bar or scoop of ice cream. From what I have been told by everyone who has experienced dumping, it only takes once. While I hope you don't ever experience the feeling, if you do, remember it will be a great behavior modifier for you.

Low blood pressure and dizziness when standing

A feeling of lightheadedness and dizziness upon standing affects around 4 percent of bariatric surgery patients. This phenomenon is called orthostatic hypotension, and it is typically a temporary, although frustrating, condition. You can experience dizziness due to a lack of water, low sodium, an adjustment to your blood pressure medication, or an expansion of your veins and blood vessels due to chronic high blood pressure.

What happens to your body to cause this dizzy feeling when you stand?

When you stand from a laying or sitting position, your body does a lot of things really quickly. I'm going to simplify this explanation so that if you are among the 4 percent affected by this condition, you'll have a better idea of how to deal with it. Let's start at the heart, where blood is pushed out to transport oxygen to all the parts of your body. When you stand up quickly, blood quickly drops toward your legs and feet due to gravity. To compensate for this, your heart rate increases to help push the blood back up. Simultaneously, the muscles surrounding the blood vessels constrict, pushing the blood back up toward the heart and brain. This system works well in most people who are well hydrated. That is, there's enough blood in the system so that the heart can easily pump blood through the body, and there's enough water in the system to keep pressure on the walls of the vessels and veins so that when they are compressed, the blood can travel against gravity.

How can you avoid this?

The key to controlling the dizziness is to keep yourself hydrated. If you are one month from surgery, there is a good chance that if you're experiencing this dizziness, it's because of a lack of water. When you are dehydrated, the volume of blood is reduced, and this puts less pressure on the blood vessels. So when you stand up quickly and your muscles contract to push the blood back up, there just isn't enough internal blood pressure to compensate for the blood that rushes down to your legs. If this is the case, drinking more water throughout the day is a good start. You may also want to drink a small amount of salty liquid, such as pickle juice, to help improve your hydration. For many people, simply increasing the amount of water they drink will reduce or solve this dizziness problem.

Another factor could be a medication you're taking, particularly a high blood pressure one. Unlike other obesity-related issues that disappear soon after surgery, your high blood pressure may take a few months to come down. If you are on blood pressure medication and it has been a few months since your surgery, talk to your doctor about your medication dosage—it may need to be adjusted now that you are losing weight. One more possible contributor to the dizziness could be obesity itself. If you have high blood pressure and high water retention, this combination could be affecting how well your system can compensate for the drop in blood pressure when you stand up. Chronic high blood pressure can increase the diameter of your blood vessels and veins, similar to how your skin will increase in size to accommodate excess body fat. So when you lose a lot of weight as well as the excess body water that comes from obesity, your system is a bit out of whack. That is, the blood vessels can sometimes take a long time to shrink back to their pre–high blood pressure size. During this time this excess space effectively reduces your blood pressure. So while drinking water and adjusting your medication are still important, you may just need to allow your body time to readjust to a lower pressure.

Nutrition

What do you eat now?

The first six weeks after your surgery is all about healing and reintroducing your digestive system to solid foods. There are typically four stages that you move through to get you back to "normal" eating. Each stage follows the standard progression of your body healing. Following is a basic guideline of what your menu for the first six weeks post-op may look like. The descriptions of these different phases are fairly general to give you an overall idea of what the stage looks like, so make sure you speak with your surgeon or dietitian about the specifics for your six-week menu.

Stage 1

Stage 1 typically starts and ends during your hospital stay. It is the shortest stage, lasting from twenty-four to forty-eight hours, and focuses exclusively on clear liquids that are low-calorie, sugar-free, caffeine-free, alcohol-free, and free of carbonation.

Stage 2

Stage 2 starts after you are released from the hospital and lasts about two to three weeks. This is when you start your reintroduction of food. But due to the trauma that your stomach has undergone, your meal choices will be limited to very soft or liquid foods. At this point in the healing process, your rule should be smooth foods (no chunks) that tend toward the bland side. Foods like plain yogurt, small curd cottage cheese, clear broth, and mild hummus will be your main go-tos. If you need some flavoring, stick to fine-grained salt and pepper only. Strain out any chunks of meat or vegetables from any soups you may want to eat. Egg whites are a good choice during this time; just avoid the yolk. The yolk contains most of the fat in the egg, and the fat can make you feel sick.

Since your food intake will be very limited, you may need to supplement with a few protein drinks or powders to get your recommended protein each day. Continue to drink water and other non caffeinated, sugar-free clear liquids whenever you need them. As a note: it should become easier and easier to drink water during this phase of healing. If at any time it is becoming more difficult to drink, contact your surgeon's office. This is going to be a difficult phase when it comes to eating. There is a chance you will quickly become tired of this limited menu, driving you to expand your diet too soon. Avoid doing this. Your stomach is in a very delicate condition, so it will not take much to damage it at this stage of your healing. You may not feel like anything is happening when you push your diet choices too quickly, but that doesn't mean it's safe to eat those foods yet. There are two ways that advancing your diet too quickly can stall or reverse your healing. First is by eating more solid foods too soon after surgery, which forces the stomach walls to expand beyond their capacity and puts significant stress on the still-healing incisions. Second, because peristalsis (the contracting and relaxing of the stomach to mix food) doesn't stop after surgery, your stomach has to work harder to break down solid foods during the first six weeks or so postsurgery. This puts further stress on the incisions.

Stage 3

Stage 3 starts around three weeks after your surgery and lasts two weeks. By this time you should be able to add a few more foods into your diet. Given your limited menu in the first two stages, this is an amazing transition. You can add extra-thin shaved deli meats, cheese, and flaky fish like tuna or sardines to your menu. Continue avoiding spicy or strongly acidic foods like hot peppers and tomatoes. Go ahead and add fruits and vegetables, but avoid anything that has small bits, like broccoli florets or strawberry seeds. Again, these smaller bits can slow down or reverse your healing. Since you are now able to eat protein in solid-food form, start to reduce the number of protein drinks you have in a day. It can be difficult to reduce the amount of protein you're drinking and still consume the minimum amount of protein you need, but the goal is to get 90 percent or more of your protein from solid foods by week six. It might help to plan your meals in advance, concentrating on packing in as many protein-rich items as you can.

If you're still having a hard time getting enough water, continue to drink as needed to keep yourself hydrated, even with meals. On the other hand, if you feel your water consumption is good, you can start working toward limiting or removing it from your mealtimes. It is a good way to start rebuilding that habit you started before your surgery. Try not to use a straw with your water drinking at this point. A straw can introduce extra air into your pouch and can have negative effects on its healing. It probably won't feel very good either.

Stage 4

Stage 4 is the final two weeks of your food reintroduction process and starts four to six weeks after your surgery. It's when you can slowly start adding in more solid proteins like chicken, red meats, and chunkier stews and soups. Start this stage slowly, introducing one or two new foods into your diet a day. Many people say that these denser proteins sit heavy in their new stomach. One way to avoid this feeling is to eat slowly by chewing your food more.

At the six-week point, your stomach should be mostly healed, so there are no major restrictions on your food choices. Yet you should continue avoiding carb-heavy foods like rice, pastas, and breads, which can create a paste-like substance that makes swallowing difficult. These foods also tend to promote gas and bloating.

Continue to add foods to your menu slowly. At this point, you shouldn't be relying on liquid forms of protein to hit your goals. Instead, focus on solid foods. If you drink your protein as your meal, you'll open the door to eating more frequently than you should, and this will add more calories to your diet, and eventually more weight to your body.

Multivitamins, fiber, and calcium

With the limited amount of food you are able to eat at each meal, you will have to supplement your diet with vitamins, fiber, and calcium. Typically these supplements are added into your diet at the six-week point in your recovery.

Taking your multivitamin daily is extra important if you've had the gastric bypass or the duodenal switch. These tools bypass a large percentage of your small intestines, where macro- and micronutrients are absorbed, significantly limiting the amount of vitamins and minerals you will get from your food source. While the sleeve doesn't have the same issues around malabsorption, the limits it imposes on the amount of food you can eat makes getting the right quantity of vitamins, fiber, and calcium difficult.

Note: Since there is no governing oversight on multivitamins, the quality of the supplements on the market is all over the place. When looking for a multivitamin, make sure to check the label to see that it's bariatric friendly; this type should give you a complete dose of each vitamin as well as making the multivitamin easier to swallow. When it comes to your post-bariatric-surgery life, there are a few vitamins that you need to make sure you're getting enough of, including the following:

B1. Helps digestion as well as contributes to healthy skin, hair, and liver.

B12. Contributes to building new blood cells and keeping your central nervous system healthy. B12 combines with a protein produced in the stomach and is absorbed in the last part of the small intestine. The tool's modifications to the stomach and intestines will affect the overall absorption rate of B12.

Iron. Iron is initially absorbed in the duodenum, but with the gastric bypass and duodenal switch, the duodenum is bypassed. This gives the body less chance to absorb iron that comes from food, which can increase the chances of a deficiency. Iron supplementation isn't necessary for everyone; a blood test can tell you if it's something you will need.

Vitamin D. For calcium absorption to take place, there also needs to be a significant amount of vitamin D to help that occur.

Calcium. When it comes to calcium, choose calcium citrate instead of calcium carbonate. While calcium carbonate is higher in calcium, it needs to be taken with food, and it needs the acid of the stomach to dissolve and absorb. Calcium citrate can be absorbed on an empty stomach with less chance of constipation. The downside to calcium citrate is that the pills contain lower-quality calcium, so you need to take it two or more times daily.

Fiber. Given the limited space in your stomach and the need to focus on eating protein at each meal, getting enough fiber from fruits and vegetables becomes very difficult. Yet you still need fiber daily for good gut health. This makes taking a fiber supplement very important. If you have lived a low-fiber life until now, start slowly; taking too much fiber too quickly can bring on bloating and constipation. The best way to introduce fiber into your diet is to start with a quarter of the recommended daily amount and slowly increase that amount over three weeks. Also abstain from starting your fiber supplement until after your stomach has completely healed to avoid any pain or discomfort. Nutritional guidelines suggest men under fifty years old should be getting 38 grams of fiber daily and 30 grams for those over fifty. Women under fifty years old should be getting 25 grams of fiber daily and 21 grams of fiber daily for women over fifty.

Specifics for the duodenal switch

Vitamins A, D, E, and K are all fat soluble, meaning they break down in fat. If you have undergone a duodenal switch, you are only absorbing an average of 20 to 30 percent of the fat you are eating, making it difficult for your body to absorb and use these vitamins. To prevent deficiency, the American Society for Metabolic and Bariatric Surgery recommends all duodenal switch patients get 10,000 IU vitamin A, 2000 IU vitamin D, and 300 mcg vitamin K daily. In addition, some duodenal switch patients will need to take an additional amount of B12. These are universal recommendations, so talk with your doctor or dietitian about the specific quantities you may need.

Iron and calcium

If you are taking an iron supplement, look for a multivitamin that does *not* include both calcium and iron because calcium will inhibit the absorption of iron in your body. Instead, take calcium supplements separately and space them out from your iron intake by at least two hours. In addition, look for a multivitamin that will be easy to swallow, either in chewable or fast-dissolving forms, or try a multivitamin patch. Stay away from gummy-style multivitamins since many of them will not have all the vitamins and minerals you will need. Gummy-style multivitamins may also have sugar as an additional ingredient.

Exercise

Starting exercise

There are several schools of thought about when to start exercising after your surgery. Some say you should wait six months or more before you start, while others don't attach a time limit but feel you need to work on your mindset before you start. And some, including me, advocate starting to exercise as soon as you are cleared to do so by your doctor. Most patients are typically cleared by their doctor six to eight weeks after surgery.

Each surgeon will have their own timeline for how long they want you to limit your exercise and movement, so take what is here as a guideline. Your surgeon's recommendations outrank this advice.

But you can start some form of exercise even during the healing phase. In fact, as a matter of good habit-building, you should start exercising during your healing phase. Keep it very light. Some rules to keep in mind during this time: For the first three weeks, at minimum, limit the amount of twisting you do in order to minimize the strain on your incisions, and for the first six weeks, refrain from lifting, pulling, or pushing anything over 15 pounds (6.8 kilograms). Given those limitations, the focus should be on cardio, mostly in the form of walking. While there is no general rule about how much you should walk daily, listen to your body. It will give you a good indication of what you should be doing. Soon after getting home from the hospital, expect the walks to be slow and quickly fatiguing. Knowing this, choose routes that are near your house so when and if you fatigue, you're not stranded too far away.

Sometime around week three of your recovery, walking may become easier, and you may be able to walk farther. This is great, but don't let this newfound ease trick you into pushing yourself too fast. You may find that on a few walks you start to push yourself to go a bit farther or faster. Be careful: your head and your body are not in the same place. Your head will want you to go farther, but your body just isn't able to keep up. Be good to yourself at this stage. When you feel like you want to go farther, use that as a sign to actually stop and go home. You may want to consider logging your walks on a calendar or with an activity monitor to ensure that you don't make too great of a leap too soon. If you are increasing your walk pace or distance by more than 10 percent each week, then you may find yourself in over your head. If you do find yourself out on a walk and realize you've pushed it too far, make sure you have your cell phone so you can call someone to pick you up. Stubbornness and valor are oftentimes rewarded with injury, and when you're injured you can't walk.

Typically, around your third week of healing, your external incisions should be closed and fully healed. If this is the case, ask your surgical team if you can be cleared for light swimming. This is a great addition to your walking, but remember to start slow. Swimming will take more energy than walking and can wipe you out fast. By six to eight weeks after surgery, all your internal and external incisions should be completely healed, and you should be cleared from your weight lifting, pushing, and pulling limit.

How you should start your workout program after you've been cleared to exercise is mentioned in more detail in chapter 8 and the bonus section on building your workout program.

Mindset

Buyer's remorse

Often people who have had bariatric surgery feel a sense of regret, or buyer's remorse, soon after the surgery. If you find yourself wondering what you've done or feeling overwhelmed after your surgery, it might help you to know that you're not alone in these feelings. Other people also have these negative thoughts and emotions. And it's natural: you've just made a significant, and more than likely irreversible, change not only to your body but to the entire way you live your life. Buyer's remorse indicates regret. It's a feeling that's ingrained in us: although we are wired to be satisfied with our decisions, sometimes we have doubts and experience cognitive dissonance. Our expectations and the results don't align. What you thought was a good decision now feels wrong. Trying to get those two sides to match up can bring about that dissonance, or buyer's remorse.

For a lot of people in this position, buyer's remorse sets in when they have completed their quest to have the surgery. Art Markman, PhD, of The University of Texas at Austin, identified this trend and calls it the *approach motivation*. Basically, before the surgery you put a lot of energy and hope into planning, researching, and budgeting. You're motivated and eager to get going with a new approach. But a few days or a week after the surgery, you find yourself dealing with the consequences of the purchase—maybe some pain, perhaps anxiety around eating or impatience for healing. You're not yet seeing the full benefits, and that makes you wonder where the benefits are. In the case of bariatric surgery, though, there is no going back. It's very natural to have that "What did I just do?!" thought. The good news: For a large percentage of people who undergo bariatric surgery, this buyer's remorse goes away fairly quickly. Most of my clients have told me that they had a day or so just after surgery where they experienced this. Yet as the pain and discomfort of the surgery starts to fade and some of the positives of this tool start to show up, like the reduction or cessation of high blood pressure, reversal of their type 2 diabetes, etc., the regret disappears. If it lingers, talk with your support group or your therapist.

The three-week stall

At around the three-week mark from your surgery, there's a good chance your weight loss will stall. It can be a bit disturbing. You've been enjoying a rapid and massive weight loss since the procedure, and it's been amazing to watch the weight just drop off. Then comes that first time you step on the scale and the number is the same as it was the day before, and the day before that. Your happy train crashes to a stop. And even though you've dealt with the buyer's remorse, it can come back with this first stall. You might find yourself thinking, "Is this it? This is all I get? What a waste of time and money! This is just like all the other diets that I've tried. This is never going to work."

But stop yourself there. Don't get too anxious about this. This is a well-known time for a stall, and most people who undergo bariatric surgery experience it. While research offers no real understanding of the reason for this early stall, think about it: You have undergone a fairly significant change to your internal plumbing followed by significant weight loss. Your body might just be taking a moment to catch up with all that has happened to it. Your best bet is to keep doing what you are doing, and ignore the stall as best you can. It may take a few weeks, but your weight loss will resume.

How you see this surgery affects your long-term success

How you define this surgery in your mind will define how successful you are at losing and keeping the weight off. The mindset that has tripped up many people in the past is that they see it as the end of living with obesity. Mentally, you've placed yourself at a finish line, with the medal already around your neck, and you believe you no longer need to do all those stupid diets and workouts, that all the work is behind you. You're done, finished, and all you need to do is go home and enjoy the fruits of the surgery's labor. These thoughts are seductive, especially if you are just so tired of being obese and want to be done with it. And the tool will help convince you that you're done, too. You won't be hungry, and the scale will show you have dropped weight and fast. But this doesn't last. Sooner than you want, things slow down. Your weight loss will become much slower or may even reverse. This can happen because you quit working on your weight loss the day after surgery. Since you thought you were finished with being obese, your mind has closed to the idea of further effort. Feeling finished stops you from continuing. If, on the other hand, you think of this surgery as a starting point to something new, then you are setting yourself up for long-term success. In a way, it's a more difficult position to be in. You will need to accept that there is a lot of work ahead, that even though you are losing weight, you still need to put in the work to get the results you want. But with a starting-line mindset—one that sees the surgery as the real starting line—this work won't be scary or intimidating: it will be exciting. You are starting a new journey in life.

An even better mindset to have for this journey is to think not of one but two starting lines. You cross the first starting line when you begin to implement the rules of the tool. This could be before your surgery or soon after. This first stage can take several months or more than a couple of years to complete. Getting these new habits down while you live in a world and a head that hasn't changed can be a struggle. Yet putting the work in and keeping on top of things will pay off. The second starting line is more fluid and less obvious, but it's there. It's there after you have spent the time and energy to integrate these new rules and habits into your life. It's there when you start noticing that you've made water a priority where before you never drank water. It's there when you go from "I *have to* work out" to "I *want to* work out." It's there when you start discovering unhealthy thought patterns and put in the work to change them. This is the starting line that puts you on the path to the life you want. It is the true starting point. Yet moving between the first and second starting lines isn't easy. You are going against decades of habits around what, how, and when you eat, drink, and exercise (if that is something you did at all). You will be changing your life, but other people in your life will be the same—and sometimes will want you to stay the same. There will still be temptations and challenges to face around food and drink. But you have motivation on your side. Coming out of this surgery and seeing the weight come off, having more energy, and feeling less pain in your daily life will help push you forward on the right path.

Take this motivation and use it. Trial and error is your friend. Experiment with different ways you can integrate these rules of the tool into your life. Reach out to others in your support team who are further along on this journey to get ideas on how to make these changes. Also know that not everything is going to work for you—and that's okay. Remember this is a journey: you will make mistakes and wrong turns. You will also have that "demon mind" that won't just disappear: it will take some time to tame. I talk about this a bit more in chapter 9. Take these mistakes and demon-mind thoughts and learn from them.

Use these lessons to keep pushing for the second starting line. By having this starting-line mindset, knowing and expecting you'll need to do some work, then putting in that work over the long haul, you will set yourself up for long-term success.

Chapter Summary

Nutrition

Eating will be weird during these weeks of healing. At first, your food will be nearly baby-food consistency. You'll likely get tired of this quickly, but it's necessary to let your stomach heal. As you get further out from your surgery, you'll add more solid foods and a greater variety of foods into your diet. Remember to go slow: your stomach is still healing, and it doesn't want to work too hard now. Keep your water intake up, and make sure you are getting the protein you need.

Exercise

Walk. Walk as much as you feel comfortable doing. But pay attention to your body, and don't let your brain bully you into doing more than you can physically do. During this healing phase, you are limited to how much you can push, pull, and lift (no more than 15 pounds), so keep any strength training to a minimum or not at all for now. If your incisions are healing well, you can try swimming around week three. This is a good time to look for a gym and personal trainer (or exercise buddy) as well.

Mindset

There are some really big changes that happen to you fairly quickly after surgery. Some will feel good. Your weight will come off fairly quickly right from the start. Losing between 20 and 60 pounds in the first six weeks is not unheard of. Also, many people who were on diabetes and/or high blood pressure medication may no longer need them. These positives will boost your motivation to keep going, and you should use this to keep building the good habits you will need for the rest of your life. The first few days after surgery can be difficult, though. Dealing with postsurgery pain, hormonal changes that stem from the adjustments to your plumbing, and a loss of any appetite—these can bring on buyer's remorse and second-guessing of your decision. Yet these feelings should go away quickly, and then you'll get to see all the good things that come from weight-loss surgery.

Chapter 8: Post-op: The First Three Months—Now What?

You've made it through the surgery. You've made it through the six-plus weeks of recovery and food reintroduction. You are probably very motivated and focused on getting this right, and you should use that motivation to your advantage. But if you are going to succeed at this weight loss, you cannot just wing it. You need to have at minimum an outline of a plan as to how you want to get to your goals. This chapter gives you some great suggestions on how you can put a plan together that works for you.

If the pillar of exercise is the weakest one for you, the exercise section gives you some great reasons to put consistent exercise into your life. This section also gives you guidelines around how much exercise you should be doing. And if you don't have a plan around your exercise, you can review the bonus content on planning your exercise. This bonus content will answer many of your questions and will give you a great starting program.

One of the most important things you can do when it comes to eating right is to have a plan around your meals both at home and when you are dining out. The nutrition section goes into more detail about all of that.

Mindset planning can be the most important and the least straightforward to implement. The sections go into detail about some of the more common mindset and habit traps you may encounter. After reading that section, you may find one or more mindsets or habits that resonate with you. If that is the case, then plan some time to work on those. That could be anything from journaling about how you exhibit that mindset in your daily life, to finding resources online to help you better understand and navigate out of those mindsets, to hiring a mindset coach or therapist to help guide you through that discovery and change of those mindsets and habits.

Taking the time to build and follow a plan that is detailed and specific to your needs will give you a significant boost toward your long-term success on this journey.

Exercise

Planning your exercise

Why is it important?

You may be asking: "Why should I exercise? The surgery is going to give me the weight loss I am looking for." After investing so much time, emotion, effort, and money into the surgery, you have a lot of faith that the procedure alone will give you the results you are looking for.

And yes, in the short term, you could probably not exercise and you'd still see some great weight-loss results. But the goal is to build a healthy new life, which includes but is not limited to weight loss. If you go back to chapter 3 (the three pillars) where I talk about the reasons exercise is important, weight loss is just one (minor) aspect among many. But don't take my word for it. Instead, let me throw some research at you.

One study from 2012 found bariatric surgery patients who consistently exercised lost almost 8 pounds (3.6 kilograms) more weight than people who exercised minimally.[19] Another study showed that patients who were active before or became active after surgery had a significantly larger increase in weight loss, with those who were active losing on average 116 pounds (52.5 kilograms) compared with those who were inactive, losing an average of 102 pounds (46 kilograms) after one year.[20]

This same study found that bariatric surgery patients who exercised regularly maintained their weight loss for at least two years after surgery.[20]

Researchers found that patients who exercised consistently lost almost 30 percent more fat mass and gained 8 percent more lean body mass after eighteen months.[21]

In this same study, participants who exercised showed a significant increase in lean body mass (muscle) over the group of nonexercisers. This showed that the first six months following surgery are critical for building lean body mass. [21]

Increased aerobic exercise or strength training has been shown to reduce depressive symptoms significantly.[22, 23]

Exercise can affect your choice of healthier dietary preferences and regulate your food intake. [24]

Research also shows a significant improvement in active people's health-related quality of life: with improved physical functioning, reduced body pain, better overall general health, and improved mental and emotional health.[25]

If you weren't already convinced that you need to have consistent exercise in your life, I hope you are now. But how do you go about doing that? Should you do it on your own or hire a professional? The answer to those questions comes down to a trade-off between time and money. With some time and effort, you can build your own workout program. Yet if you don't have the desire or time to put into building your own workout program, then hiring a professional to do that for you is a better way to go. Either way takes some planning and time. If hiring a personal trainer, you will need to spend some time finding and interviewing a few people before you hire them. If you've decided to build out your own workout plan, then there are some questions you will need to answer in order to build something effective. With either route, if you are feeling a bit lost on how to start, the bonus section on hiring a personal trainer or building a fitness plan will give you plenty of information to get you started. Though before you commit to either of those paths, you need to take a little time to clarify what you want from your workout time. Why are you working out? What are your goals? This will help keep you focused on what's important to you, giving you the drive to continue when motivation wanes.

The "why" in your workout

I've already said that exercise is important for preserving muscle mass and helping with weight loss. So there are two good reasons to work out. But these reasons are general and apply to everyone. You need to find a reason that is personal, a reason that really speaks to you, a reason that will get you up off the couch and to the gym when your motivation is low. You need to find a reason that sparks your desire to keep going even if it's just small steps. The answer is probably very similar to your reasons for getting weight-loss surgery in the first place. And if it's not, you can start with those reasons as you look for your personal exercise motivation. I'll give you an example.

Mary is a longtime client. Before her surgery, Mary told me she was taking multiple insulin injections daily, and it was taking a toll on her. She just couldn't do it any longer, and this was the primary reason she'd decided to undergo the procedure. But the thing that made her most nervous wasn't the surgery itself—it was having to exercise. She had never done it and had very little confidence that she could. But despite never having gone to the gym before, and despite her lack of confidence in herself once she got there, she was in the gym consistently. What got her there was her "why." It was that very strong desire to never again take another injection of insulin. More than a few times she told me that "exercise is tough, but it's still a thousand times better than all those injections."

Mary knew that exercise was helping her build muscle and boosting her overall weight loss. Both benefits were important to her, but they weren't what got her to get up and head to the gym. That motivation required her personal why—no more insulin shots. This is the kind of thing you need to find for yourself. It's a reason you can lean on when the motivation isn't there; it's what you can refer back to when things get tough and you'd rather skip the workout for the day. It doesn't matter what this reason is, as long as it resonates on a deep level.

If your "why" isn't as obvious to you as Mary's was to her, then start with a simple statement: "Why am I exercising?" Whatever the answer to that should lead to another "why" question until you find something that feels personal and real to you. Here's a short example of this:

Q: "Why am I exercising?

A: To build muscle mass and help with my weight loss.

Q: "Why do I want to build muscle mass and lose weight?"

A: To be healthy and strong (or at least not skinny and weak).

Q: "Why do I want to be healthy and strong?"

A: To be able to interact with my kids more and not feel worn out so fast.

Q: "Why do I want to interact with my kids and not wear out?"

A: I don't want to miss out on their lives because of my weight and unhealthy lifestyle.

When do you stop asking why? When you *feel* the right answer. You'll have an emotional connection to that reason. In the example I just provided, playing with the children is important—but this reason goes to a deeper level than just playing tag or catch with the kids. It's being able to create a strong connection, to bond with them, to show them love and to be personally happier because of it. That's the "why" in this example. Your "why" answer could be completely different, but as long as it has a strong feeling associated with it, then it's a good answer. You want a "why" strong enough to help you on those "I don't feel like it" days. If you can tap into this feeling, it can help you put on your gym clothes and start moving. So the stronger you can make your why, the better it will motivate you.

This feeling doesn't have to be positive either. The final answer to Mary's "why" was based on a fear of going back to a life that made her miserable. It was this fear that drove her to continue with something that she, at first, didn't enjoy but knew would get her to a better place. A part of questioning yourself on your "why" should include asking, "What happens if I don't do the work?" Taking time to imagine your life if you decide to not do the work may push you more than imagining your healthier future. Humans naturally move away from unpleasant things. So by tapping into that negative feeling of what it would feel like to not do the work, you may find yourself in the gym and cooking healthy meals more often.

Take a little time to figure out your "why." That's your motivation. Once you have your "why," you will want to be effective with your workouts. In the next section, I go over the basic guidelines for what your workouts may look like.

Basic guidelines for beginning workouts

You may be all in to exercise into your new life, but the question then becomes, what does that look like? Here are a few general guidelines that can get you started.[26]

- Your exercise program should consist of both aerobic and strength training.
- For the exercise to be effective, you should be doing 250 to 300 minutes of moderate to intense physical activity each week.
- You should be strength training three to four days per week, alternating days between cardio and strength.
- When starting your strength training program, you should have between six and ten exercises, doing between twelve and fifteen repetitions for one to three sets.
- To make your strength training effective, you should be eating 1.5 grams of protein per kilogram of your ideal body weight.

If working out is new in your life, these guidelines can seem ambitious. Don't let that discourage you; here is a progression you can follow that will get you to these numbers.

Exercise progression during first year postsurgery

After you're cleared by your doctor, you should start walking. (I went over this in earlier chapters, so I'll do a quick review here.) During the first six weeks after surgery, you'll want to walk as much as your body, energy levels, and time let you. Your doctor will advise you on limitations, likely telling you to lift, push, or pull no more than 15 pounds (6.8 kilograms) at a time to avoid damaging your incisions and sutures. But after you've been cleared by your surgeon, you can do much more.

Six weeks to three months

If you are new to exercise, start with either bodyweight exercises or use the machines in your gym with a very light load. If you are new to strength training, start slowly: two or three thirty-minute sessions each week should be enough to get your muscles feeling tired without overtaxing them. As thirty minutes becomes easy for you, start adding in fifteen more minutes to each session until you are doing an hour a few times a week.

For cardio training, pick up where you left off during your healing phase. Slowly increase either the time you spend doing cardio or the intensity with which you do it. Your goal should be to do between three and five hours of vigorous cardio a week. Have one or two rest or restorative days each week.

Three months and beyond

If you have been consistent with your workouts, you will notice around three months after you started some big improvements with both your strength and cardio. This is a good time to start reevaluating your plan. If you haven't changed much with your gym routine, modifying your workout will help you continue to challenge muscles and cardiovascular strength. As you continue, your body will start adjusting to work, and you will be able to safely change one of your rest days into a workout day, but you should always have a minimum of one rest day each week. Refer to the bonus content if you want a more in-depth discussion of how you can set up a workout plan.

What can you do if a gym doesn't work for you?

Sometimes the traditional forms of exercise won't work for you. This doesn't mean you don't have options; there are other non-gym ways to build strength and cardiovascular health. Here are a few you may want to investigate:

- Swimming
- Aqua aerobics
- Walking
- At-home workouts
- Online beginner-friendly yoga

Or if movement is difficult, especially near the beginning of this weight loss, look into SilverSneakers. This program is primarily built for an older population, but because of this, many of their classes are gentler and beginner friendly. This can be a great way to step into exercise in a way that isn't intimidating or overwhelming.

Nutrition

Planning your meals

As you begin to reintegrate more foods into your diet, you'll discover a lot about how your modified stomach works and what you can and can't tolerate. Though it's possible that these tolerances will change over time, there often will be instances where certain foods you were able to eat before your surgery just don't agree with you anymore. This phase of your post-op journey can very much be about trial and error, where you are learning what works for you, what foods you can and can't eat, how to integrate any specific guidelines that your dietitian gave you, and what happens when you go rogue from those guidelines.

One common outcome of this surgery is that your sense of hunger will be reduced due to how this tool affects your hunger hormone. While this feeling may not last forever, it's in the first three months to a year that many patients report an odd "hollow" feeling instead of hunger. I bring this up to help you understand that you will need to be more deliberate about your eating habits in the first six to twelve months. Your hunger will come back to some extent, which will add in new challenges around eating, but for these first few months or so, you need to be very strict with yourself around your nutrition and water intake. You may think not having an appetite is a good thing, but without that natural cue on when to eat, you can find yourself behind on your daily protein and water intake. This may not seem like a big deal, but not keeping up with your meals can have many negative effects, one of which is slowing or stalling your weight loss.

If you start to notice this happening, one solution is to set alarms during the day to remind yourself to eat and drink. It can be annoying, but if there is no effective internal cue, you will need to make an external one. If your schedule is such that you have very little time to sit and eat a meal, then you need to make sure you always have a quick and easy source of protein. Protein bars, cheese sticks, or nuts can help you stay on track with your weight loss, though these shouldn't be considered a full meal. When you don't really know what to do, go back to the rules of the tool. They will guide you on what you need to do to be successful. This next section is focused on giving you hints and tips around some of the more common trip-ups that can occur in these first three months.

How to bring foods back into your life

Around six weeks after your surgery, you will be cleared to include any food in your diet. But just because there are no more restrictions around foods you can eat, you neither can nor will want to eat certain foods.

Ease into "new" foods

In chapter 5 we talked a lot about how your senses of taste and smell will change after surgery. You will quickly find out what foods you can tolerate and which foods are no longer on your menu. This change in your taste can make you hesitant to try new foods, especially if you are eating out at a restaurant or a friend's house. Yet it doesn't have to be stressful. Following are some suggestions on how to approach different restaurant menus and meals cooked by friends without sacrificing your goals.

Dining out

At some point in your journey, you will want to go out to a restaurant. You may feel excited—but also nervous because your control over what you can eat will be limited. But plan ahead, follow these suggestions, and you'll be fine.

- Check out the menu before you go. Most restaurants post menus online. Take a look and

128

plan your meal; if you're worried that the menu may have changed, have a backup choice.

- Because you can eat only a limited amount of food, you may find the appetizer and side dish menus are more suitable than an entrée in terms of volume. Use caution if you try to order from the children's menu—it's often filled with meals that are fried, carb heavy, or fat laden.

- Share a plate with a friend. This is a good, fun option, but if the restaurant is picky about this, let them know about your surgery. If you're not comfortable talking about it, you can say that you have a limitation with how much you can eat. Most good restaurants will accommodate your needs. (Some surgeons give patients a "bariatric patient card" to show servers at restaurants, which requests smaller portions or to allow the bearer to order from the children's menu. Remember that restaurants don't have to honor those cards and have a plan for it.)

- Ask your waiter to bring a to-go box out with the meal so you can put half (or more) away before you even start your meal.

- Ask to have carb-heavy and starchy foods (french fries, potatoes, rice) replaced with vegetables.

- Choose proteins that are baked, grilled, or broiled; avoid breaded or fried foods.

In addition, here are a few specific choices you can make in different styles of restaurants. When you face down the menu, remember the rules of the tool, and repeat this mantra: baked protein, vegetables, and light on the starch.

Fast food

On the whole, fast food isn't a great choice for anyone. But if you do find yourself at a fast-food place, choose the grilled chicken option and remove the bun. If that option isn't available, pick a bunless hamburger. With any option, if the meal comes with a sauce, ask if you can have that on the side to help reduce the amount of calories.

Italian and pizza

Pasta and pizza are many people's favorite foods, and that can make finding something that suits your tool a challenge at these restaurants. If you're eating pizza, go for a thin crust (or cauliflower crust, if possible), and choose toppings that are mostly lean proteins and vegetables, like grilled chicken or roasted peppers. Some people even just eat the toppings from a slice of pizza and find that satisfying enough.

As much as it pains me to write this, I advise that you use a knife and fork to eat your pizza. Cutting it into smaller pieces and eating it slowly can reduce the amount you eat. If you go with something other than pizza, make it a meal that avoids heavy cream sauces and includes quality lean proteins. If the dish is noodle heavy, eat the protein first and have just a few bites of the noodles at the end of your meal.

130

Asian

Asian restaurants are likely to have a good selection of foods you can choose from, though it's a good idea to stay away from noodle dishes like lo mein and pad thai as they are heavy in carbohydrates and sodium. As with any restaurant, choose a protein that hasn't been fried or breaded, like tempura. Tofu, shrimp, and grilled chicken are all good choices. Again, since your meal will be small, choosing an egg roll or a spring roll and eating just the filling would be a good way to go.

Family-style and bar food

If fried foods are a trigger for you, it's best to stay away from family-style and bar food restaurants, but that's often easier said than done. These restaurants usually have a large menu of foods; this has pluses and minuses, so you'll need to be disciplined when you order. These restaurants usually have a large selection of appetizers and kids' meals, and you can stick to these for portion control. When possible, go with a grilled protein like chicken or fish. If you choose a burger, order a basic patty, limit the condiments and toppings, and only eat the meat. Avoid starchy and simple-carbohydrate foods like french fries and rice, or substitute these with steamed or broiled vegetables.

Mexican

When you're looking at a menu offering the American version of Mexican food, it can be difficult to find a meal that isn't heavy on cheese and sauces. The best go-to here is the fajitas—you'll get grilled steak, chicken, or shrimp along with vegetables. Just skip the tortillas. If you choose a burrito or enchilada, focus on the fillings more than the tortilla, and in particular focus on the protein more than any other part of the meal.

These are just a few of the types of restaurants that you may find yourself in, but you'll notice a repeated pattern: focus on quality lean protein, and avoid simple carbohydrates and grains in favor of vegetables. As for dessert, the choice depends on how sensitive your stomach and taste buds have become to sweet foods. In addition, there may not be that much space left for a dessert to begin with. Yet if that is an option, you'll want to choose a fruit option or something small.

Another situation that might come up is a meal at a friend's or relative's house. If you've told your hosts about your surgery and new way of eating, that can make it easier: you can talk with your host about the menu before the date and either ask for an adjustment or, better yet, test the food beforehand. If you're not comfortable talking about your surgery and food choices and asking for an adjustment isn't an option, here are a few things you can do:

- Try eating before you go: you can still sit with your friends and maybe eat something small.
- Eat only the protein that is served and push any sauce off to the side.
- If it's a buffet, use a smaller plate and choose mostly protein.
- Chew your food slowly, and really pay attention to your fullness level.

How many calories should you eat in a day?

Daily calorie intake is a logical concern since every weight-loss program under the sun talks about calorie reduction. Yet with bariatric surgery things are different, and counting

132

calories isn't as important, especially the first year post-op. If you hate counting calories, this way of eating should feel more freeing and less of a burden. If you like to count calories, then you may want to work on breaking that habit because this isn't a typical weight-loss program—it's a new way of life. And part of this new life focuses on building habits that follow the rules of the tool, plus knowing—and trusting—that your stomach size and reduced hunger will control your calorie intake for you. So instead of focusing on calories, you should be focused on getting enough quality protein daily (minimum of 65 grams) and drinking enough water (48 to 64 ounces daily). As mentioned, it is more important to know the volume of food you are eating at each meal rather than the number of calories that meal gives you. Yet if you still need to know how many calories you should eat daily, then the following chart gives you a range you can work within.

Surgery timeline	Calories	Protein (g)	Carbohydrates (g)	Fat (g)	Fiber (g)
Pre-op diet	900–1,000	60–90	<50	<50	15
Phase 1 post-op diet (0–1 week)	<100	<15	<10	0	0
Phase 2 post-op diet (2–3 weeks)	450	60	<20	<10	4–8
Phase 3 post-op diet (3–5 weeks)	400–600	60	<20–45	<10–20	10
Phase 4 post-op diet (5–7 weeks)	600–750	60–70	<45–50	<20–25	14
Phase 5 post-op diet (7–9 weeks)	800–900	60–80	<75	<30	17
9 weeks–6 months post-op	850–950	60–80	<90	<30	17

1 year–18 months	1000–1250	70–80	<90–120	<40–45	20
Active (250–500 calories/workout)	1400–1600 female 1800 male	80–95 female 100 male	<135–155 female <210 male	<60–65 female <80 male	20+ female 25+ male

Always choose complex carbohydrates in the form of fruits and vegetables and focus more on good fats like avocado to get the healthiest options. But if you are hitting your daily protein number and following all the rules of the tool closely, then the tool will limit your overall calorie intake, and you shouldn't have to worry too much about counting calories.

What you may have noticed with all these suggestions is the amount of planning you need to do around your meals. Whether it's scheduling when you can drink water (refer to chapter 4 for an example of a water drinking schedule), scheduling your meal breaks, or planning your meals (your macronutrients, volume of food, restaurant choices), there is a lot that goes into this process. Don't let it frustrate you. You don't have to do it all at once. Remember, this is a long journey and a big change in how you will live your life. If it takes a while to get all of this under control, that's okay—just keep working at it. The more that becomes second nature to you, the more successful you will be.

In addition to building up your eating and drinking habits, there are a few things to be aware of around foods— in this case, sugar alcohols and artificial sweeteners as well as how alcohol affects you after your surgery.

Sugar alcohols and artificial sweeteners

Sugar alcohols are naturally occurring sweeteners that create the sweet taste of sugar in sugar-free foods. There are four common sugar alcohols: sorbitol, maltitol, xylitol, and erythritol. Each of these has a slightly different and reduced sweetness intensity compared with natural sugar. Sugar alcohols also have a slightly lower calorie count than sugar, which makes them a primary choice for food manufacturers. Another positive aspect of sugar alcohols is that they don't promote a spike in insulin as sugar does, and they also help prevent tooth decay. Yet all these good things come with a downside for many people, especially people who have had weight-loss surgery. Because most sugar alcohols don't get absorbed into the bloodstream, they stay in the digestive tract, which can promote diarrhea, gas, and bloating.

Erythritol is an exception since it is the only sugar alcohol that is mostly absorbed into the bloodstream and removed through urine, reducing the typical side effects. However, since each sugar alcohol is less sweet than sugar, they are often combined in sugar-free foods, making it challenging to find products with only one of these ingredients. Artificial sweeteners, such as saccharin, sucralose, aspartame, neotame, and acesulfame, are also used in many low-calorie foods and drinks. Like sugar alcohols, they can cause bloating, gas, nausea, and diarrhea. While not universally accepted,[27] some research shows an increase in abdominal fat and a greater BMI than people who do not regularly consume artificial sweeteners.[28, 29] Therefore, incorporating or continuing to use artificial sweeteners in your diet may hinder your overall weight-loss goals after bariatric surgery.

Alcohol after surgery

You should strive to keep away from alcohol as long as possible after your surgery. As a matter of fact, you should refrain from any alcohol for a minimum of six months after surgery, with twelve months or longer being a better goal. There are some good reasons for this abstinence. First, alcohol offers calories but no nutrients. This alone should be a reason to limit your intake or just avoid it altogether. If that doesn't motivate you to keep the alcohol in check, you should know that the surgery itself can change how your body deals with alcohol.

When you drink beer, wine, or any liquor, your body starts to break down the alcohol in your stomach via an enzyme called gastric alcohol dehydrogenase. The longer the alcohol stays in your stomach, the more it breaks down. This leads to a smaller amount of alcohol entering your bloodstream. After bariatric surgery, especially gastric bypass, the smaller stomach significantly reduces the amount of this enzyme, as well as the time the alcohol stays in your stomach.[30] This reduced time in your stomach means more alcohol goes into your bloodstream, which increases the overall effects of the alcohol. For bariatric patients, this increase in time and intensity of alcohol is more than an interesting fact. Studies show that this change in alcohol metabolism can have a negative effect on some people's ability to regulate their overall alcohol consumption.[31] In addition, there is a population of weight-loss surgery patients who have a greater tendency toward alcohol use disorder (AUD). This population is mostly younger males who had AUD, smoked, and/or had a drug habit before surgery. Research into bariatric surgery patients and alcohol use shows that alcohol consumption usually stays low in the first year post-op, but a small yet significant portion of the post-op population picks up or returns to an unhealthy use of alcohol a few years after surgery.[32, 33] These studies show that this trend is more significant with people who have undergone gastric bypass. Part of this increase in alcohol dependence could be attributed to the fact that gastric bypass promotes faster absorption of alcohol into the bloodstream, which will make you feel more intoxicated. One result may be that some people seek this feeling more often, especially if they experienced a similar feeling from eating in their presurgery days. In one study of over 11,000 participants that compared gastric bypass with lap band patients, individuals who had the gastric bypass procedure showed an increased risk for higher alcohol use than those who'd had the lap band procedure.[34] This can lead to a transfer from one addiction—food—to another—alcohol—which is talked about more in the next section.

Mindset

The first three months after your surgery, you will start to see some big changes, both physically and mentally, in your life. It can be challenging to navigate all of this, so in this section, I want to highlight a few mindset traps and habits you can incorporate into your life.

Let's start with the one habit you need to get right before you can tackle any other issues, and that is paying attention to *you*.

Mindfulness: paying attention to you

The word *mindfulness* has been used a great deal over the past few years, and for many people, it has lost its meaning. If you are one of those people, let's change the word for you. When you see mindfulness, think paying attention because that is generally what it is. It's paying attention to you, how you react to things around you and emotions that come up in you, and how they make you feel, physically. Paying attention is the foundation of all things that go into changing habits, whether they are physical, like eating and exercising, or mental, like how you think about yourself, how you set boundaries, or how you interact with others. I bring this up specifically because many people live a reactionary life. They act in ways that have no thought behind them. It's like living in a fog—you don't know where you are and only act when you bump into something. On the other hand, being more mindful (paying attention), you understand who you are, what you do, and how you react to things in your life; it's lifting that fog from your life. It's awareness of all things in and around your life. Being mindful is reflecting on your actions, it's being aware of your emotions, how those emotions make you physically feel, and understanding what brought those emotions to the surface. It's understanding your relationship with others, creating boundaries with others, being able to connect with others on a deeper level because you are aware of your needs and can articulate them. So how does all this mindfulness stuff help with your weight loss? Not to be too dramatic about it, but ignoring yourself, the probability that you will lose the weight you need to lose and keep it off is close to zero.

An example of this comes from a client who five years ago hired me as soon as she was cleared for exercise. She worked with me for about six months, was hit or miss with showing up for her sessions and doing her "homework," as well as not following the rules of the tool. One day I got an email from her telling me that she was going to stop working with me, and she fell off my radar. Five years later, I got an email from her asking to start working out with me again. In those intervening years, she had gained all her weight back and then some. She had only contacted me because she was going in for a revision. A few years after she quit with me, she started working with a therapist who helped her become aware of who she was and what she was doing that sabotaged her weight loss. It became clear that she had an eating disorder, one that she never really saw. In her mind, that was only something skinny people had, not her. But by becoming more aware of herself, she was able to see what she could never see before. It was because of this work of lifting the fog around her life that she was able to understand why she initially failed with her weight loss. It was only then that she had the confidence to go in for a revision and genuinely put in the work needed to be successful.

I am using this one story of many as a cautionary tale. As you go through this journey, you *need* to be aware of you, what makes you tick, and what areas you need to work on.

Addiction transfer, or cross-addiction

Addiction transfer is when one addiction is limited, but the underlying issues that created that addiction are not addressed—so another addiction will take its place. This secondary addiction can be most anything; shopping, sex, drugs/alcohol, smoking, gambling, and exercise are a few possibilities. Within the world of weight-loss surgery, there is a prevailing idea that addiction transfer will occur in this group more often than with other populations. This belief comes from the fact that a larger percentage of people who've undergone bariatric surgery have a food addiction, and that when food is reduced, another addiction will take over.[35, 36] But there is no strong evidence that transferring a food addiction to some other addiction is more prominent with bariatric surgery patients.[37] This isn't to say a new addiction can't take hold after surgery. As mentioned, there can be a tendency of people with the gastric bypass to increase their alcohol intake due to the increased absorption time of the alcohol and the more intense feeling they get from alcohol. There is also a study that shows a small increase in nicotine use a few years post-op.[37] It could be that this transfer of an addiction is associated with someone who has shown a history of certain risk factors, such as:

- Binge eating or compulsive eating.
- Drug or alcohol addiction, including cigarette smoking.
- Avoidance of working on past traumas.
- Bouts of anxiety or depression.

If you have one or more of these risk factors, that doesn't mean you will definitely move from one addiction to another. But knowing this and becoming aware that it may happen will possibly help you avoid an addiction transfer. If you are unsure if you may be starting to develop a different addiction to replace a food addiction, the following list can help you start to sort it out—or better yet, talk with a professional about your concerns.

- Experiencing anxiety, depression, or suicidal thoughts whenever access to the transferred addiction isn't possible.
- Losing a job, home, relationship, or friendship because of the addiction.
- Obsessive thoughts about how to gain increased access to the object of the addiction.
- Health problems related to the addiction.
- Money problems directly caused by the addiction. [38]

Whether addiction transfer is a big issue or not, it is wise to be aware that it could happen. And again, if you are concerned about it, talk to your doctor or a mental health professional.

Don't compare yourself with others

It can be difficult to see or hear of weight-loss successes that other bariatric surgery patients experience when you don't see the same success. It's important to remember that you cannot match their journey to yours; the only data points that should be meaningful to you are the ones that come from you. I know it's easier to read than to practice, but working on your own journey is important. You don't have to do it on your own—nothing could be further from the truth—but you do need to personally understand your needs and limitations and be able to address them. It's these needs and limitations that are unique to you that makes any comparison to others fruitless and possibly harmful. If you are a fifty-year-old comparing your weight loss to that of a thirty-year-old, then you are going to find some big differences. Age plays a big factor in weight loss, even with bariatric surgery. Your metabolism is different, your endocrine system is different (hormones change as you age), and you may have injuries and movement limitations. You may also be in different phases of life when it comes to your career and family, and this can play a big role in your weight loss. Even if you are of a similar age to someone else, there can be big differences in how and why people lose weight. What you can do is start to get to know yourself better. This can include what exercises you like and will do consistently, how you can work around any injury with your exercise, what foods you can enjoy, and how your body responds to those foods. Know how your work and family life will affect this journey, and know who your support team is and what they can provide.

It's also good to get to know people who have had success. Asking them what they have done—both successes and failures—can give you new ideas to try, better ways to do things that were not working well for you, or permission to stop trying things that don't work at all. For your own journey, it's all about where you are now in comparison to where you were. Sometimes one small change will keep you going; things like this are known as nonscale victories. When you start paying attention to these, you can feel a positive difference in your motivation and mindset around this journey. The next section talks a bit more about this.

Celebrating nonscale victories

Nonscale victories (NSV) are just what they say they are: any positive change that isn't a change of numbers on a scale. These are the "little" things that change during your weight loss that can provide a huge and positive boost to your mental well-being. It's easy to let them pass by or not give them much thought, but being aware of them and even celebrating them a little can add more motivation into your journey.

 Some of the more common NSVs that show up with weight loss are:

- Fitting into a certain pair of pants for the first time in years.
- No longer needing a belt extender when flying.
- Easily fitting into a chair with arms.
- Not being out of breath after climbing a flight of stairs.
- Being able to get down and up from the floor without much effort.
- Confidently taking a bath.
- Sleeping without a CPAP machine.
- Reaching healthy levels in your blood work.

- Having more energy.
- No longer having joint pain.

This list could go on and on, but the idea is that you should look for the small things that have changed in your life due to your weight loss that make it easier. Take a few moments to appreciate these changes—maybe write them on your calendar or in a journal or keep a list on your phone. By keeping track of these victories, you'll have a history of your progress that isn't weight related, and in some ways, this is a more important metric of your success.

Emotional eating: non hunger reasons people eat

In earlier sections we discussed eating slower taking a specific amount of time and taking time to chew your food. This was all about keeping you from wanting to eat between meals. Those are good habits to work on and will help, but hunger isn't the problem when it comes to emotional eating. Emotional eating is about soothing and/or avoiding difficult situations or over celebrating more positive situations. It's something that happens on autopilot. It's old programming that helped you cope in the moment but now isn't helping.

So how do you approach this situation? First, if you feel this is a big issue for you, then looking for a mental health expert who has experience with emotional eating is a good place to start. In addition, start becoming more aware of when you eat but are not truly hungry. Body hunger is a slow progression and over the course of an hour or so becomes more and more pronounced. Head hunger (emotional hunger) shows up much faster, with a craving for a particular type of food. Typically, emotional eating is triggered by a specific emotion or emotions, usually, but not always, associated with unpleasant feelings. Eating is a way to avoid the feeling and the discomfort that comes from it. For some, it's something learned from an early age.

During one of my sessions with a client, we were discussing emotional eating. She had told me that emotional eating had been a part of her life since she was six years old. From her own admission, her family life wasn't very happy or stable. Her parents had frequent and loud arguments. After the fights ended, her mother, with good intentions, would give my client ice cream or chocolate to apologize for the yelling. Over the years, sweets became her go-to when she found herself in similar situations. Most of the weight she gained happened while working for a verbally abusive manager. After being yelled at by her manager, she would hit the vending machine for chocolate and go back to her office and eat it all. It was only years later, working with a mental health professional, that she made the connection between eating and yelling.

If this story sounds familiar to you, there are some actions you can take to help you avoid going directly to food when strong emotions come up. Before going directly for the comfort food of choice, try one or more of the following:

- If the desire to eat is coming from a stressful place, take some deep breaths. Controlled breathing is known to lower your blood pressure and stress level.[39]
- If you can, do something physical. Go for a walk, do some squats, dance, fidget. Anything that gets you moving will help preoccupy your mind and work out any stress.
- Write in a journal about anything, talk with a close friend, or sing or talk it out with your pet or plants (they won't mind).

- Plan ahead. If you know you are going to be in a stressful situation, think of things besides eating you can do in advance that can help you.

Since we are talking about emotional hunger, once you start to stabilize your emotions through one of these suggestions or something else, you will notice that your desire to eat will have lessened as well.

Other Things That Happen in the First Three Months

Hair loss

Many people worry about losing their hair after bariatric surgery. While there is no way to completely avoid hair loss after bariatric surgery, the good news is that the loss is temporary, and if you put a bit of preventive measures in place, you may limit the loss.

Why do you lose hair after surgery?

The type of hair loss that comes from bariatric surgery is called telogen effluvium. This is when the body transitions more of your hair out of the hair growth cycle and into the shedding cycle, so that you lose hair before new hair has started to grow. With this process, hair loss increases three-to-five-fold over normal daily loss. Telogen effluvium usually starts about three months after surgery, but the condition usually corrects itself within a few months. The exact reason for this is unknown, but there is strong evidence that the abrupt change in your diet, along with the reduction in the nutrients absorbed after surgery, are the reasons for this hair loss.

What can you do to slow the hair loss?

There are a number of options you can try to help with your hair loss. Unfortunately, there is no one or two things that are going to guarantee a reduction or prevention of your hair loss. But the following options are a good place to start.

Eat enough protein. Hair strands are made up of protein fibers, so when your body is not getting enough protein for all its functions, one of the first places your body looks for spare protein is your hair. When this happens, you'll notice that your hair becomes more dry and brittle. Dry, brittle hair can increase the overall loss. You can reduce the chances by eating enough protein daily.

Get a sufficient amount of vitamins daily. Biotin is the most frequently suggested vitamin to reduce hair loss. Yet there is little conclusive evidence that biotin can slow or stop hair loss. Biotin's importance comes mostly from increasing the rate of new hair growth. And since surgery can bring on telogen effluvium, taking biotin can reduce the amount of time for new hair to replace the lost hair. Foods that naturally contain biotin are egg yolks, whole grains, and meat. Vitamin D is known to, among other things, help stimulate new hair follicles. With a lack of vitamin D, new hair growth can be limited. There is some limited research showing that supplementing this vitamin can help reduce the effects of telogen effluvium.[40] There is evidence that people who have telogen effluvium also have low iron levels.[41, 42] Yet the jury is still out on whether low iron levels affect hair loss. Some studies found some benefit in iron supplementation in people with low iron levels and a reduction in hair loss,[43] while some studies found no clear association between low iron levels and hair loss.[44] What this all means is that if you are taking an iron supplement for low iron levels, it may help with your hair loss, but it probably shouldn't be your only path to slow the loss. Zinc is an essential mineral that cannot be created in the body and has to be supplied through foods. There are mixed results concerning the effectiveness of zinc and hair loss. Research shows that gastric sleeve patients reversed hair loss by increasing their zinc intake.[45] But conflicting research shows no improvement in hair loss with a zinc supplement.[46] If you feel strongly about your hair, you might try zinc and see if it makes a difference for you.

It is difficult to avoid the loss of hair that comes from bariatric surgery, but it usually is short lived. Keeping up with your multivitamins, getting enough quality protein daily, and getting tested for an iron deficiency can help reduce the loss of hair overall.

Excess skin: what you can do about it

One of the main concerns after bariatric surgery is the excess skin that remains after you lose so much fat. There is no way to completely stop this from happening. As your body continued to store fat, your skin expanded to accommodate the excess fat cells. When you rapidly lose fat, your skin has a difficult time returning to your pre-obese size. How significant your excess skin will be and how much you can slow or prevent this sag has a lot to do with your age, genetics, how well you eat, whether you are a smoker, and how much sun damage you have had over the years. The procedure that you have will also affect the amount of skin sag; the duodenal switch results in the most skin sag.[47] This isn't surprising, since the duodenal switch is also the procedure that produces the most weight loss.

What influences your skin's elasticity?

Your skin has three main layers: the epidermis, the dermis, and subcutaneous. The dermis is responsible for your skin's elasticity. It holds collagen and elastin. Collagen is a tough protein that strengthens your skin and keeps it durable, while the protein elastin helps the skin stretch and spring back to its original shape. Obesity compromises the quality of both of these proteins, reducing the skin's ability to rebound after your weight loss. While your skin will bounce back somewhat about a year after weight stabilization, depending on factors of age, genetics, previous skin care habits, and the number of years you've been holding on to excess body fat, this could be a limited reduction of sag.[48]

Based on the evidence of obesity's negative effect on skin's collagen and elastin, there really isn't much you can do to stop the sag. But keeping well hydrated and exercising can help.

Hydration. Skin cells need water to be able to do their job well. When you are dehydrated, your skin becomes dry and flaky. This lack of water reduces your skin's ability to bounce back from being overstretched. While there is little direct evidence that drinking water will hydrate your skin, water is the main pathway to help replenish skin cells.

Exercise. You have probably read that exercise can help keep your skin from sagging after surgery. I wish this was the case. While exercise helps with keeping your skin healthy and functioning by increasing blood flow to the skin, the reason for the sag isn't a lack of exercise. There is a myth that circulates on many blogs and message boards around exercise and its ability to "fill" the sag with muscle. You can't just add the same amount of muscle that you lost in fat—you'd need to add more muscle than the fat you lost. By volume, muscle takes up about four-fifths of the space that fat does. While technically you could fill the space with muscle, it wouldn't be an easy or fast activity. You can lose 8-plus pounds a month in fat from this tool, but even with very dedicated strength training, you may be able to add just a pound or two of muscle in that same time frame. This makes the amount of work you'd need to do to fill the void left by fat to be unsustainable for most people, and not really even necessary. This isn't to say that you shouldn't try to build muscle: you should. But the goal behind your muscle building shouldn't be about filling the space where body fat used to be.

Skin-removal surgery

Many bariatric surgery patients consider this option at some point in their journey. The surgeries that are available to you depend on what parts of your body you want to have the excess skin removed from. For many people, the most common surgery involves removal of the excess skin around the lower abdominal area. This excess skin is commonly known as the pannus, or apron, that hangs over the thighs and genitals. This procedure is called a panniculectomy, and its goal is to remove this excess skin with very little body sculpting or modification of underlying musculature. Good candidates for a panniculectomy have a pannus that makes activities like walking or exercising difficult; they may have difficulty keeping these areas clean; and they may have sores and rashes that are difficult to treat due to the excess skin. Usually due to the inability to keep this part of the body clean and healthy, insurance companies may cover some or all of this procedure.

Another type of skin removal is called a circumferential body lift. It recontours the body around the skin-removal site, which the panniculectomy does not do. This surgery removes excess skin and reshapes the areas around the lower abdomen, upper thighs, and butt. Since this surgery doesn't fix a medical condition but is a more cosmetic treatment, most insurance companies don't cover this procedure. This surgery can cost from $6,000 to

$20,000 depending on the complexity of the surgery, location, and skill of your surgeon.

If you are planning on either of these procedures, there are few prerequisites that must be met before you are able to have the surgery. Your surgeon and possibly your insurance company will want to know that:

- You have maintained a stable weight for a minimum of six months.
- You have no preexisting medical conditions that would prohibit the surgery.
- You understand the outcome of this surgery—there will be scarring.
- You're not planning on getting pregnant after surgery, as it can compromise the results of the procedure.
- You can take six to eight weeks to ensure full recovery.

If this is a route you would like to take, the process of finding a surgeon is the same procedure you used to find your bariatric surgeon (revisit chapter 2 for more details). Take time with this and find a surgeon who will do the best work for the price you can afford.

Chapter Summary

Exercise

Having exercise in your post-op life is not optional, and while it will enhance your overall weight loss, its importance extends to all aspects of your health. How you decide to exercise, whether it's with a personal trainer or building your own program, is up to you. Having a specialist can offload much of the program building around your fitness routine, and they can help you start to really understand proper form and good overall movement. Yet hiring a qualified trainer can be a big hit to a budget, so if you are going to go that route, take your time to interview a few different people so you find someone who is going to fit your needs. If you decide to go it alone, take time to build a program that works for you and that continues to be challenging to you. While it can be less expensive than a qualified trainer, it can take more time to get everything right. But if you follow the program building in the bonus section, it can reduce a lot of frustration.

Nutrition

The first three months post-op are the time to put all that pre-op habit-building you did into practice. Making sure you are drinking enough water, eating protein at each meal, measuring your food volume, chewing your food more, etc. In addition, having a plan around eating when you don't control the menu, like at restaurants and dinners at friends' homes, can really help you stay on track. These first few months are also a time of discovery around what foods you can and can't tolerate, including sugar alcohols and artificial sweeteners. All of this can be overwhelming and strange at first, especially the lack of hunger and change in your taste. But go at it slowly and treat this start of your new life as a time of discovery of who you are changing into.

Mindset

This is going to be the weirdest time for you in this journey. I say that because of all the changes that start to show themselves during these first few months. You'll be dropping weight quickly, changing how you look. You may experience envy around other people's successes as well as envy toward you from people still struggling with their weight. You may notice that people start to treat you differently, which can bring on both positive and negative reactions. With all these changes, the one big takeaway from this time is to not be tough on yourself, to be mindful of what you're thinking and doing. Seek out support to help you through these significant changes. As time goes on, you will start to feel more comfortable in your new body, both physically and emotionally.

Chapter 9: Post-op: The Second Half of Your First Year

This is the last phase of your first-year post-op, and at this point in your journey, you should be seeing a significant reduction in your weight and increase in your energy level. You may also notice that there is still a long way to go, yet it's all about adjustments and giving yourself the opportunity to experiment more with activities. But trying these new activities can bring out the "demon mind," which is always trying to tell you all the things you can't do. There are a few other worries that can start to show themselves at this point in your journey as well. You may be able to eat more food at each meal, which can bring up a fear of whether your stomach has expanded. You may notice that you are not losing as much weight as some other people, or that you are stuck or further from your goal weight than you want to be. And a big change that starts to show itself as you start to lose more weight is the change around your relationships with other people as well as with yourself.

This is also the time you are starting to step up to your second starting line. I brought up the idea of two starting lines previously in this book. The first line starts as soon as you say yes to the surgery, and the second line starts as the changes you've made over the past year become more commonplace in your day-to-day life.

Exercise

Start trying new things

If exercise has been a fairly consistent part of the past six months or more and you've noticed that the progress around your strength and cardiovascular fitness has started to level off, it's a good sign that you need to change things up. I go into more detail about this in the bonus section, but I'll give you a brief overview of what I am talking about.

Your body needs to be challenged consistently to make changes, grow muscle, and become stronger. Your body is also doing its best to be as efficient as it can be, so after a few months of consistent exercise, your body will start to level off its growth of new muscle and strength. To combat this, you will need to plan changes into your long-term fitness program. It could be more or fewer reps and sets, it could be adding new movements and formats, or it could be adding new activities. Since I go over the first few changes you can make in the bonus section, I want to focus on the last change here: adding new activities.

One general complaint about exercise and working out is how boring it is. While this can be true, it doesn't have to be. As you get further and further out from your surgery, you will have lost more weight and found it easier and less painful to move your body. When this starts to happen, you need to take advantage of this change by experimenting with new activities and forms of exercise. The purpose is to experience many ways you can exercise and hopefully find an activity or two that you enjoy doing. It's when you connect with the activity on an emotional level that it stops being about having to exercise and more about wanting to exercise. At a deeper level, when you find an activity that you truly enjoy doing, it no longer feels like exercise at all; it's just something you do because it makes you happy.

It can feel overwhelming at first to go down this route; you may have no clue what you would like, and that's okay. If this is the case, cast a wide net. Try every activity you can find. Try all the group classes at your local gym, try various styles of yoga, try cycling, running, hiking, walking, swimming, rock climbing, martial arts, etc. There is a big chance that you will not like most of them, and that is part of the reason for doing this—to narrow down what you do enjoy doing. At the same time, the more activities you try increases the chance that you will find one or two you do enjoy. It's these activities that you should give your time and attention to. You will probably feel uncomfortable and awkward at whatever it is you want to pursue; that's just the nature of being a beginner. Yet the more you do the activity, the more you will improve and in turn, the more you will enjoy doing it.

Secondarily, when you find an activity you enjoy, you may start looking for other exercises and workouts to help improve your skill and strength in the activity you love doing. Embrace this opportunity—it's something you probably didn't have the ability to do in your presurgery days. As an aside, if you really want to get the most from this experiment and truly get a taste for how these other activities feel to you, I would suggest first taking a few months to work on your strength, endurance, and skills around movement. Improving your strength and becoming more aware of your body and how you move will make these new activities less intimidating to try. A good example of this came from a client who worked with me for about a year. After about nine months of working together, I started talking about her expanding her activity horizons. It took a bit of convincing, but when some new friends talked her into going indoor rock climbing, she decided to go for it. She absolutely loved it and started going a couple of times a week. To her this wasn't exercise but a fun and challenging physical activity that she never thought she would be able to do. Finding a new activity that she enjoyed doing didn't stop there; she was all in on getting better and better, and that drove her entire workout plan. Before finding this new hobby, yoga was something she never thought she would do. Now because it helps her with climbing, she never misses a class. In our sessions, we started working on movements and challenges that complemented her climbing.

This client may be an outlier when it comes to how strongly she took to climbing, but I use this example to demonstrate that branching out and finding something you enjoy doing will affect your entire mindset around exercise and working out. Workouts and classes that you may not have thought about trying become more important because they help you with your new hobby. You will also take on a more positive mindset around exercise, as it will help you become better at the activity you enjoy doing. So, take some time to find something fun.

Nutrition

Has your stomach stretched?

The question of a stretching stomach is one that worries many people who have had this tool. The idea of losing the feeling of restriction on how much they can eat terrifies them. Usually, noticing a significant increase in the capacity of your stomach takes more time than the first year, but I want to address this issue now to help you plan on how to minimize any increase that may occur. It's natural and expected that your stomach capacity will increase. Depending on how much it changes, this can be a mentally uncomfortable place. But has your stomach actually expanded? Is this fear that you just mess up this tool and negated everything valid?

The good news is that unless you have the gastric band or the stomach balloon, your stomach reverting to its presurgery size isn't going to happen. Yet after some months, it's going to get easier to eat more food in one sitting, so what is happening? Initially, your stomach's capacity is fairly small, and it doesn't take much food to feel full. As you get further out from your surgery, the amount of food you can tolerate at any meal has a lot to do with your eating and drinking habits. This is part of the reason for the rules of the tool: to keep guardrails around these habits. If you start straying from these rules, the more it feels like your capacity for food increases. And while there is some physical increase in the overall capacity of your stomach, a lot of this increase comes from how sensitive your stomach is to the expansion from food.

The feels of your stomach

What makes you feel full is the communication between your stomach and your brain. As food enters the stomach, there are stretch receptors around the stomach that react to this increase in the size of the stomach wall. As more and more food enters the stomach, these receptors send a stronger and stronger signal to the brain until there is a tipping point. This tipping point is when you feel that full feeling stopping you from wanting to eat more. The sensitivity of these receptors changes with your eating habits. The consistency of your meal size will set a baseline for what your brain considers full and overfull. If you are concerned about the volume of food you can eat at each meal, there is good news. Research shows that after just four weeks on a reduced food intake diet, there is a corresponding increase in how fast people start to feel full when the stomach capacity is pushed beyond its established

157

baseline. On the other hand, with people who frequently eat larger meals, the signal that goes to the brain to indicate full and overfull takes longer.[49] The conclusion from these researchers was in part that these stretch receptors become less sensitive in someone who frequently eats larger meals. While this research was on people who had not gone through weight-loss surgery, this idea that eating an increased amount of food consistently and thereby changing the signal around fullness makes sense for bariatric surgery people as well. If you go back and look at the rules of the tool, you should start to see how some of the rules (don't drink at meals, measure the volume of your food, chew and eat slowly) line up with keeping these stretch receptors around your stomach sensitive to overstretching, helping you feel full sooner. So while there are some physical changes to your stomach size after time, how much you eat may also have to do with the signals around your stomach becoming less sensitive to the amount of food you are eating.

If this has happened to you or you're concerned about it happening to you, what can you do about it? One way that people try to get back to that feeling of fullness that they experienced soon after surgery is with a pouch reset.

What is a pouch reset, and do you need one?

The idea of resetting the pouch actually came from a bariatric surgery patient who, a few years out from her surgery, wasn't happy with the increased capacity of her stomach. She thought her stomach had stretched, so she came up with an eating schedule that she hoped would reduce the size of her stomach.

The method behind the pouch reset is to mimic the first few stages of food reintroduction just after surgery. It starts with a liquid phase, moving on to a soft-food phase and concluding with the reintroduction of solid foods. This method will, for most people, restart their weight loss and will have them start feeling fuller from eating less food. This is great, especially if it breaks a long-term weight-loss plateau. But from the research summarized in the previous section, this pouch reset probably has less to do with shrinking the capacity of your stomach and more to do with resetting your "full signal." To most people, it doesn't matter if their pouch is shrinking or just becoming more sensitive—if it helps the weight loss, they are happy. The reason I bring up this distinction is to reinforce the idea that if this reset method works for you, then there is a good chance that you have not messed up your tool. Additionally, this reset can help you readjust your habits to the rules of the tool.

Before you consider doing a pouch reset, consult with a professional dietitian who understands weight-loss surgery. With their help, you can get a more focused and personalized plan that will be more successful. Also, if you have any specific dietary needs, they can help navigate those issues before you begin.

Mindset

Approaching your second starting line

The second starting line is when you are able to start settling into a new routine and integrating new habits around eating, exercise, and mindset work into your daily life. So how do you know when you are approaching your second starting line?

One way to know you're getting there is when nonscale victories become commonplace. As I mentioned before, a nonscale victory is when you discover that you can do something that in the past was unthinkable—

activities like jogging up a flight of stairs, crossing your legs, getting in and out of a bathtub, or instinctively reaching for a glass of water. When you first notice these changes, it's exciting and motivating, and it is something you should celebrate. When that activity becomes something you just naturally do or expect without really thinking about it, that's when you know you have entered a new part of your life. When a friend asks you to do something active, like go for a hike or walk around a museum for a few hours, and your first reaction isn't fear about how your weight will stop you, then you have reached a second starting line. When you are not surprised about being able to walk up a few flights of stairs easily, then you've started your new life. When joint pain that was attributed to your weight disappears for good, then you've started your new life.

Just as important, there are nonphysical indicators of reaching the second starting line. One of the biggest is an acceptance that this weight-loss journey will succeed. That it's not a diet that will fail like all the rest but a complete change to your life. An example of this came from one of my clients, who told me a few weeks before her one-year post-op anniversary that early on she didn't trust that this was going to work. Even after losing 50 pounds in the first five months, she wasn't convinced. She had lost 50 pounds twice before (albeit not that quickly) and both times ended back at her starting weight. For her it was only after breaking that 50-pound-loss barrier and maintaining that loss would she be convinced that this was different. She did see that loss increase, and at the end of her first year, she was down 85 pounds and becoming happy with the changes that were happening. She was seeing that the eating and exercise habits she had been building over that first year were becoming easier to commit to. What were once exciting nonscale victories were becoming commonplace in her day-to-day life. Her life had truly started to change for the better, and she knew this was something that would last. She had reached her second starting line around her acceptance of this being more than a diet.

What you may have noticed is that this second starting line isn't as definitive as the first starting line. When my client reached the starting line of accepting this procedure as more than a diet, she still was working on integrating other habits into her new life. That's how this second starting line works. You will start living a different life around some parts and will still be moving toward your second starting line in other parts of your life. That's perfectly acceptable, it's just how life works. Yet the more you work on building good habits, both physical and mental, the sooner you can start more and more of your new life.

If you are not where you want to be, that's okay

Reaching your second starting line doesn't mean that you are "done," and you may even feel frustrated at not being where you want to be. One issue that my clients often mention is that they don't feel like they are where they thought they would be after so many months. Usually, this stems from unrealistic goals and expectations that either they set or were set for them about how much weight they can lose. Some surgeons give their patients an idea of what their final weight should be. It's not meant as a rock-solid goal weight but an estimate, from their professional experience, on what could be achievable. The weight-loss surgery itself can give you a skewed vision of your future final weight. It's easy to want to upgrade your weight-loss goals and timetable for achieving this loss when you start seeing your weight coming off. But remember that this rate of loss is short-lived. That a slowdown in your weight loss is expected and is healthy. Sometimes you may have based your weight-loss goal number on another person's results, maybe someone who has lost a lot of weight and looks great. This was discussed in more detail in chapter 8 on not comparing yourself with others. It's easy to want to emulate their success and model your goal on theirs. But you're a different person, and you will respond differently to the weight-loss efforts.

If you have found yourself discouraged about not hitting your goal weight, remember your reason for setting that particular goal number. Ask yourself if it was meaningful to you, or were you using suggestions from someone else or examples of other people's losses that were ultimately not achievable for you? Additionally, if you have been set on a specific scale number as a sign of your success, then you have limited your idea of success. There are many parts of this journey other than the scale that you can use to measure success. The section later in this chapter called "Your goal weight isn't important" goes into more detail as to why you shouldn't put too much emphasis on the scale number.

Yet one thing that can get in the way of building less weight-related goals is the demon mind. It's a mean little voice that can be difficult to silence. It's the "voice" or feeling you have when you look in the mirror and wonder if you are worthy of your new weight. It's the times when you fall back on the idea that you are too fat or too out of shape to do some activity. You know it's a false thought, but it's still something you have to battle.

How do you beat your demon mind?

So, how do you beat your demon mind? Don't listen to it. Yes, I know that is a glib answer and sometimes much easier to read than it is to do. Yet I have seen many of my clients win their battles with their demon mind time and time again. Two such clients stand out to me as good examples of people who achieved significant goals while fighting this little demon.

Getting to the top of a mountain

A client of mine wanted to summit one of the 14,000-foot peaks here in Colorado. It was something she had thought about for a few years but never truly believed she could do because of her weight. We had been working together for a few months before she told me about this goal, but she didn't feel it was achievable. That is, her demon mind was telling her she wasn't capable even though she had already lost a significant amount of weight. But we talked about it, and she decided to take on the challenge, reasoning that even a failure to reach the summit was still a success because she had never done it before. But her demon mind didn't let go that easily. After nine months of work and additional weight loss, she had the strength and the ability to reach the summit, but she wasn't there mentally. Her demon mind was telling her she couldn't do it. I didn't push it; we just kept working on the program I had built for her. It was during one session she told me she was sick of putting it off and decided it was time to attempt the summit. We planned the hike, met at the trailhead, and started hiking. She made it to the summit and back. She told me that while the climb to the summit was difficult, convincing herself she could do it and not listening to her demon mind was much more difficult. That before the hike she was so nervous that she was very close to canceling the hike completely. But she looked back over the past year of work she'd done to get to this point and knew she could do it. After that day, she told me that her demon mind is a lot quieter than it used to be. Today she still goes on difficult hikes regularly and easily takes on other activities that once would have been unimaginable.

One hundred miles on a bike in one day

Another client had a son who was training to ride a century (one hundred miles on his bike in one day). My client wanted to do the ride with his son. For my client, just telling me that goal was difficult because his demon mind kept telling him, "That's ridiculous, you'll never do that." What made it even more challenging was that he had not been on a bike in over twenty years. We started slowly, first focusing on basic fitness, building good habits, and working on dropping enough weight to feel comfortable on a bike. His demon mind was still strong, keeping him from seeing the gains he was making. But as he saw the weight come off, he became more confident about getting on the bike. It was a slow start, but after a few sessions of bike riding outside he told me that his demon mind, which was telling him he couldn't do it because he was "too fat," was becoming quieter and quieter. His confidence grew alongside his fitness, and sixteen months after his surgery, he completed his first century ride. When I asked him about it later, he admitted there were certain parts of the ride where his demon mind almost got the better of him, telling him he couldn't do it. But he persevered and crossed the finish line. The reason he says the demon mind didn't win was because he knew he had put in the work, that he had trained, ate well, and wasn't living his old life anymore.

While over the course of time both of these people reached their second starting line when it came to integrating new activities into their lives, it wasn't always easy for them. There were many times when self-doubt got the better of them, times when they let their demon mind talk them into bad decisions around eating or not exercising. What kept them going was that even when they allowed their demon mind to take over, it was always temporary—and they knew it. They always came back. They were consistent. It wasn't easy for them, and I don't expect it to be easy for you either. But being good to yourself and not letting your demon mind continue to define who you are will allow you to achieve things you would otherwise think impossible. You don't have to climb a 14,000-foot mountain peak or ride one hundred miles on a bike to quiet your demon mind. Yet working toward something you find challenging with consistency and persistence—and doing it—will go a long way toward quieting your demon mind.

Your goal weight isn't important

Deciding that your goal weight isn't important can seem strange to a lot of people who are trying to lose weight, whether through bariatric surgery or in a less invasive way. But it's true: your weight, those numbers on the scale, shouldn't be your main goal when it comes to weight loss. There's a lot more to it than hitting an arbitrary number. And since your weight can fluctuate 4 or 5 pounds in a day, trying to maintain a certain weight can be difficult and unproductive. In addition, if you've put a lot of pressure on yourself to hit a goal weight, it can be mentally draining when you come close but don't actually get there. As I have mentioned before, this weight loss is more than hitting a number. It's about building a new life, giving yourself the opportunity to do things you've never done or haven't done in a long time. That's where your focus should be, on building that life. If you are spending more time and effort basically trying to reach some number on the scale, you are missing the point.

Instead, you should be asking yourself questions about activities and setting goals related to those activities. They don't have to be running a marathon or climbing a mountain, but if you can focus on being able to walk up ten flights of stairs without stopping, play with your children more easily, or just have more energy during the day, that's a more sustainable place to be mentally. In addition, if you've been focusing on keeping or increasing your muscle mass, then chances are high that your scale number won't move much or will actually go up. If your focus is all on a scale number, this lack of change or an increase in that number can be discouraging, especially if you've been busting your butt at the gym.

       An example of this is my client, Kim. She told me at the beginning of her weight-loss journey that she was shooting for a 120-pound loss in order to reach her college weight. That was the skinniest she remembers feeling in her life. At fifteen months post-op, she was down a little over 100 pounds and had not lost much after that. This weight-loss plateau was very discouraging to her. She had put a lot of focus on that college scale-weight number and couldn't seem to get to it. The thing was, she knew why she wasn't losing much more weight. Part was due to stress at work and how she dealt with that, part was from her commitment to adding more muscle mass, and part was at this point in her journey, the weight just comes off more slowly. The combination of these factors added up to her not seeing the "right" number on the scale. It took her some time to reframe the goal in her head before she was happier with her success. Changing her focus away from an arbitrary number on a scale to more meaningful achievements helped. Looking at what she was able to do with her life now that she was down more than 100 pounds of fat reinforced in her a new definition of success. She felt, and was, stronger and more flexible, which allowed her to pursue more activities with more confidence. She was able to get into a pair of pants and a dress that she always wanted to fit into. Taking a bath instead of a shower was now something she could do easily and lifting her 75-pound dog into her car wasn't a struggle anymore. Her list went on and on in this fashion. As she started to add up all these nonscale victories, the goal of reaching her old college-day weight no longer made sense. When she refocused on what she'd gained from her weight loss, the number on the scale seemed much less important. Even at 20 pounds above her goal weight, she was much healthier than her presurgery days, and that discovery made her much happier.

Setting a goal weight isn't wrong, but it shouldn't be the most significant goal in your journey. Look for all your nonscale victories, add them together, and see if that helps change how you feel about the level of success with the weight you've lost so far.

Change in Relationships after Your Surgery

There is a popular belief that people who undergo bariatric surgery have a high rate of divorce. The good news is that this belief is not completely accurate. Recent research shows that for most people who have weight-loss surgery, their romantic relationship either stays the same or improves.[50] Most romantic relationships that fail are from underlying interpersonal issues that existed before the surgery and then surface after surgery.

While it is good news that this procedure doesn't have as big of a negative impact on romantic relationships as popular belief would have it seem, there can be some big changes that occur that, if not discussed, can strain a relationship. Let's address a few areas where you may notice some strain in your relationship.

One big thing that happens as you lose all that excess weight is your energy level increases significantly. If presurgery you and your partner were happy to be less active, that will change. Anecdotally, I've heard from many of my clients that they are surprised with all the energy they have. That it has become difficult to sit and watch television. That instead they will clean or go for a walk just to relieve that excess energy. If you and your partner were happy to spend time together in less active or sedentary hobbies, this could be a point of contention, especially if your partner is hesitant to embrace a more active life.

The relationship you have with eating and your partner may also change. If you two were each other's "eating buddies," that will definitely change. For many people, having an eating buddy can be a way to hide or lessen the guilt around binging. Yet in addition to you not being able to eat like you used to, there is a strong pull to "get this right," and this once-shared activity goes against that goal. When this goes away in one of the partners, it can strain the relationship. On the other side, you may notice a new dynamic where your partner becomes more focused on your eating, with a good intention of helping you stay compliant with your meals. Some people will find this beneficial; others may see this as a food police. While it may be coming from a place of concern and wanting to be helpful, depending on how it is approached, it can feel more judgmental than helpful.

Your sex life may also change after surgery. Obesity has a strong impact on reducing libido. After surgery and a considerable weight loss, a significant portion of this population notices an increase in their sexual desire. If your partner experiences a low libido due to obesity or some other condition, you could find your sexual relationship difficult to navigate. There can also be a sense of jealousy from your partner that other people are noticing you, or your partner may have an unexpected response to your new size. We all have preferences for what we find physically attractive, and this "new you" may not be what they find physically attractive.

Yet as I mentioned at the beginning of this section, not everything is a negative when it comes to this new life. A significant percentage of people who have this surgery report that their relationship with their partner improves. People report that they have a more positive physical

168

relationship with their partner, which brings about a stronger connection. This surgery and the resulting healthy changes that come from it can rub off on your partner as well. You may notice that they start making healthier changes to their diet and movement. They may start to exercise more and make better food choices, which in turn can strengthen your relationship.

Other, non-romantic relationships can also change after your surgery. You may notice that friends you had before surgery fall away from your life. You may also notice that new people come into your life. Depending on the relationship you have with friends, coworkers, and family, you can attempt to mitigate any issues by talking with them. But in most cases, unless they are very close to you, you may just need to let them decide what they need to do with their relationship with you. It can be disappointing, frustrating, and sad if someone you have known for a while decides your decision to become healthier is too uncomfortable for them to stay in a relationship with you. But this isn't your fault. They are the ones who have made the decision for themselves as much as you are the one who made the decision to have this surgery.

I bring up all these issues not to deter you from the surgery but to help you set expectations and to give you the opportunity to start discussing these changes with your partner, friends, and family. If you don't feel comfortable doing this on your own, look for a professional who can help guide you. Whether it is just you or you and your partner, or a larger circle of friends and family members, learning how to talk about this difficult subject can help you and the people around you navigate these changes in a healthier way.

Your Body Image

Another relationship issue you may face is the relationship you have with your own body image. This surprises many people after they lose a significant amount of weight. How you feel about yourself may not change, but how others now see you can be a surprise. A statement intended as a compliment may have an unsettling effect on you, maybe causing you to rethink your previous relationship with the person. Then there are the ideas you have about how you look. Many of my clients have told me in one way or another that after a significant amount of weight loss, they don't really know who they are looking at when they look in a mirror. They all say that this is a happy mental disconnect, that the person they are looking at is healthier and happier than what they were expecting. Yet they all say it was a surprise how long it took to accept who they had become physically.

An example of how this mental disconnect can show itself in even small ways comes from two clients who worked out at the same time with me. They had both gone through weight-loss surgery around the same time and would often discuss different aspects of their journey. One day they started talking about how after losing a significant amount of weight, they both felt they looked fatter than ever. This didn't make sense to them. They knew logically that they were smaller than before the surgery—that was obvious in many ways; but the feeling of looking fatter was still there. The more they talked about it, they concluded this feeling came from the clothing they were wearing. Before surgery, both of their wardrobes were mostly baggy, oversized dresses and shirts. Now, after a significant amount of weight loss, they were both wearing clothing that was more fitted to their body size. Their choice of clothing had "exposed" their body shape more, and they equated this exposure to feeling fatter. This discovery opened up a discussion around body image, their presurgery expectations, and what they are experiencing now. The conclusion they came to was that while their bodies were not where their pre-op expectations had them, they were very happy with where they were. The decrease in joint pain, cessation of many kinds of medications, and the ability to just move easier outweighed the feeling of being more exposed.

Body image and past trauma

In a more serious example of how body image can affect your weight loss can come from past trauma. There has been an increase in research around how childhood trauma, especially sexual trauma, increases the chances of obesity. A portion of the obese population that experienced sexual trauma are overweight as a protection against future trauma.[51, 52] This type of defense mechanism to deter future abuse can have a big effect on your body image as you start to lose more and more weight. If this is something that resonates with you, you may notice that as you get closer to a specific weight, it may become more difficult to lose beyond that limit. Some researchers call this a "barrier weight," or a weight where a trauma took place, and getting below this weight is difficult since it can feel like removing the protection they had put in place.[53] Without positive and supportive trauma therapy, it can be very difficult to get below this weight. Note: This idea of a "barrier weight" is mostly a hypothesis, and there still needs to be more study to determine if it is valid. Yet the reason I discuss this idea is that anecdotally, I have had clients tell me that working with a therapist on their trauma has had a positive effect in breaking a plateau on their weight loss. This could be associated with a barrier weight or not, but working through a trauma does have its benefits.

These two examples are the extremes of how you can react to the change in your body. That something as seemingly small as a different size shirt and pants affects how you see yourself. Or it could be that this change in size and weight can bring on a host of other issues that need to be addressed to keep you successful.

Pregnancy after Bariatric Surgery

For many people, the reason for weight-loss surgery, at least in part, is to help with fertility and increase the chances for a healthy, trouble-free pregnancy. For others, the increased fertility and libido that comes from this procedure is a little surprising and may lead to an unwanted pregnancy. This increase in fertility comes from big changes in your hormones after the surgery. In the pre-op section, I mentioned that your hormones affect your taste after surgery; something similar can happen with the reproductive system as well. In addition to a change in hormone levels, weight-loss surgery can lead to a return to normal ovulation and menstrual cycle, along with a complete resolution of polycystic ovary syndrome (PCOS), which contributes to a lack of ovulation, making conception much more difficult.[54, 55] With this dramatic change in fertility and libido soon after surgery, the chances of pregnancy can increase significantly. Yet whether you are planning on having a child after your surgery or not, most bariatric health care specialists discourage pregnancy within the first eighteen months postsurgery and strongly suggest using some form of birth control during this time.

There are a few reasons for this delay. The biggest is that in this first year, you will be losing a lot of weight through a severe restriction to your food intake. If you become pregnant in this time period, you can struggle significantly to get all the nutrients you need as well as the extra for the fetus. Malnutrition of the fetus can occur if you are not focused on your eating. This malnutrition can be more significant if you have undergone either gastric bypass or the duodenal switch, because both of these tools rely on malabsorption. Although you are strongly encouraged to keep up on your multivitamin supplements after surgery, it's still possible that you'll experience nutritional deficiencies in yourself and your growing fetus. In addition, during the first year after surgery, your body is in a prolonged state of ketosis. That means your body doesn't have enough carbohydrates to use as fuel, so it uses body fat. While this can help you lose excess body fat, there are some animal studies that show being in ketosis while pregnant has a detrimental effect on the fetus.[56] But as you start to stabilize your weight loss, your body will transition into ketosis less often, making it less of a health issue.

Another aspect of pregnancy after bariatric surgery is the psychological aspect of having to eat more (if possible) and also the weight gain involved. After you've dedicated a year or more to losing weight, this can be a difficult transition to make. Giving yourself a year or more to work on any body/eating issues can help you navigate this weight regain you will need to do for a healthy pregnancy.

While this section is focused on women and pregnancy after bariatric surgery, there are a few studies on fertility in men after surgery. Within these few studies, the results have many of the same positive outcomes as with women. One study shows that men who have undergone weight-loss surgery experience an increase in testosterone and a reduction in an estrogen hormone estradiol.[57] Yet one very small study of six men who underwent bariatric surgery showed a decrease in fertility, which the authors of the study suggest may have to do with the reduced nutritional needs for spermatogenesis.[58] Yet with such a small sample size, there is a lot of room for more study into this aspect of male infertility and bariatric surgery.

For many women and men, this increase in fertility can be another positive aspect of this surgery. For others, it can be an unwelcomed surprise, whether it's an unplanned pregnancy or a reactivation of their menstrual cycle. In either case, knowing that this surgery can change your fertility level can help you make some important family-planning decisions.

Chapter Summary

Exercise

This last six months is an amazing time for you when it comes to exercise and trying new things. Your weight is down enough that weight-related joint pain is reduced or has gone away completely. With this smaller body, you can now start to feel more comfortable with trying new activities. It's through this activity experimentation that you can find something you love to do, which can change your relationship with exercise. This ability to start doing new and different activities comes from the work you've been putting in since your surgery date. And to keep that part of your exercise routine going, you may need to start looking to change that up as well.

Nutrition

Your stomach will grow in capacity naturally as you get further from your surgery. A healthy expansion should have you eating about half a cup of food for each meal. Yet if you feel you are able to easily eat more than that, you may think you've messed up your tool. You haven't, and by taking a few weeks to eat smaller meals, you should see the sensitivity of your stomach return. Yet before you go down that route, you may find it helpful to talk with a qualified dietitian.

Mindset

The further you get from your surgery, the slower your weight loss will be. This slowing down can be frustrating, especially if you've not reached certain goals. It's even more frustrating when you attach your level of achievement to what others have accomplished. But taking stock of all that you have achieved since your surgery, the things that have changed you for the better, the weight you have lost, and the improvement of your health will help you reframe what goals are important to you. It's also a time when you and others start to see some significant changes to your body shape. As these changes become more and more obvious, relationships can start to change as well. This could be for the better or the worse, but being aware of these possible changes gives you the opportunity to help the people in your life (and yourself) better navigate all of this. These last six months can start to be a mental challenge, but if you start to work through this with a mindset coach or therapist, you can see some great and positive changes.

Chapter 10: Year Two and Beyond

Obviously, your weight-loss journey doesn't stop at the end of your first year, but it does start to take on a different focus. Whereas the first year or so is all about building habits and navigating all the changes that occur, the second and subsequent years are about establishing these habits around eating, mindset, and exercise. It's the continual work of crossing that second starting line for all three pillars and making these habits "just what I do now." Since this is a lifelong journey, the more you practice the habits to be successful, the easier they become. As this practice goes from deliberate and focused to more second nature, the ease of losing the excess body fat increases. But more importantly, by establishing these habits, you increase the opportunity to maintain your weight loss.

For well over half the population that undergoes weight-loss surgery, there is some amount of weight regain that occurs three to five years post-op. One study saw a weight regain in 56 percent of the participants. Of that 56 percent, almost a third had regained more than 10 percent of their total weight loss.[59] A different study whose goal was to see what factors contribute the most to people's weight regain found that poor dietary habits and limited physical activity were the biggest contributors to limited weight loss and more weight regain.[60] So the more you work to establish these habits of exercise, eating, and mindset, the greater the chance you have of achieving and, more importantly, maintaining the weight loss.

These following years are also about discovering all the things you can do with this new life. For many of my clients and other people I have talked with over the years, as they lose more weight and feel more "free," their goals start to change. Initially, goals around diabetes remission, lower blood pressure, less joint pain, and other health-related benefits dominate. And as these goals are achieved, the goals around getting past that second starting line (consistency with good food choices, exercise, and starting to know themselves better) can take over. Sometime around eighteen to twenty-four months after surgery, new goals start to be added. These are typically goals that at the start of this journey may have been considered "crazy," yet now they seem realistic. The stories before about climbing a 14,000-foot peak in Colorado or cycling a hundred miles in one day are an example of that. Other examples I've heard and witnessed range from competing in a powerlifting competition to a seven-day cycling tour of Vietnam. You may have a "crazy" goal or two as well. A goal that you would love to accomplish, but there is a voice in your head that says, "Yeah . . . that's not going to happen." You know that little "demon mind." But you also know that you are not that person anymore. You've made massive changes to many aspects of your life, and you have given yourself the opportunity to pursue those crazy goals.

In addition to the freedom to pursue bigger goals, the further out you get from surgery, the more this journey takes on a familiar feeling. You are no longer at your second starting line; you've passed it, and it's just your life. It's when you look at yourself in the mirror and expect to see the person everyone else sees. When you are buying new clothes, and you know your size; you don't go to the XXXL section first. When you've found a fun, active hobby, and it's just something you do and enjoy now.

All this comes from understanding and integrating the rules of the tool and the three pillars of weight loss into your day. To do this and make it a natural part of your daily life, you need to build a plan around how all this will work into your life.

Nutrition is following the rules of the tool and modifying them as needed to fit your lifestyle without watering down the reason for them. For some people, there is a give-and-take around these rules; some become part of their life, and others get modified to fit their life. These changes can slow or stall weight loss, but for some, the trade-off is okay. Exercise for a lot of people who go through bariatric surgery is at first very intimidating and foreign, yet if you've taken the time to educate yourself or hire a professional, this piece becomes one of the easiest pillars to stick to. Mindset is by far the most difficult and the most important of the three. The difficulty can come from a stigma you may have around mental health professionals. It can come from feeling that you don't actually need it. And even if you are working with a professional, the difficulty of wading through your limitations and traumas is very real. This is a dynamic journey. What you set for goals and successes early in your journey may not be what is important later. You may notice that the further out you are from your surgery that you are focused more on one of the three pillars. This isn't a bad thing, yet you may want to ask yourself if this focus is due to a need to improve in this area. Or is this focus because you know and understand this pillar more and are ignoring the others? It's from this place of comfort that you can find yourself out of balance. Maybe you're exercising more, but how and what you are eating have fallen off the radar. Or you've nailed down your eating habits and meals, but you've just never made time to work out like you should. This is what makes this journey dynamic, and it will take continual assessment of where you are, what you are doing right, and what you would like to improve to keep your success going.

Finally, I hope that this book has helped you start to see how this procedure works and what you need to do to make it successful. I hope the best for you and your weight-loss journey.

Bonus Section: Planning Your Exercise

Exercise is a nonnegotiable part of your success with this tool. Without putting consistent and progressive movement into your overall weight-loss and health plan, you will not see the success you are looking for. It's because of its importance in your journey that I have built this bonus section. This bonus section addresses the two most common paths people take when it comes to starting exercising after their surgery. You can either hire a personal trainer or build out your workout program on your own.

If you decide to hire a specialist, finding the right one is important to your commitment and safety. Yet finding that person can be challenging, especially if you are new to exercise. This next section gives you some questions to ask during your search to help you find that person.

If you would rather go it alone, there is a bit more work you will need to do. Section 2 outlines a good, basic plan that you can adapt for your needs.

Before you start your exercise program, whether it's with a personal trainer or built yourself, get checked out by your doctor. While you may find another visit to the doctor frustrating, it's critical that you know any physical limitations you may have before you start. And knowing these limitations will be beneficial to the creation of your exercise plan.

Section 1: Finding the Right Personal Trainer

Hiring the right personal trainer can significantly improve your chances of not just sticking with your workouts but also learning to actually *like* exercise. The right trainer will help you identify what you want from your workouts and what activities you may be interested in pursuing, and they will build a detailed plan to help you achieve those goals. Additionally, hiring a personal trainer can help you better understand how you move and how you need to move to be safe during your workouts. Finally, a personal trainer can keep you on track, motivated, and accountable when you are not "feeling it." Yet as with any specialist, personal trainers can be an expensive part of your budget, so if you are planning on going down this route, this section will help you find a trainer who works best for you and your specific needs.

How do you find a qualified trainer?

The research required to find a personal trainer is similar to what you did while finding your surgeon. Start by asking friends or family members. You could also ask your surgeon's office if they have any suggestions for trainers. Social media—especially bariatric-friendly sites or groups—can also help you out. Your local gyms will most likely have a population of personal trainers to talk with. If you can, try to interview three personal trainers. This will give you the opportunity to compare different methods of training and different personalities. The following list of questions isn't exhaustive, but it gives you a good place to start. If you have any specific needs, you will want to add those to this list as well. While you are interviewing your candidates, also pay attention to their personality and how they interact with you. Can you get along with this person? Do they have a similar personality to yours? Do they seem professional? Most of the time you will just know—so don't ignore your feelings one way or another. This will be someone you will be seeing a few times a week each week for months, so personality goes a long way toward you being consistent with your workouts.

Personal trainer interview questions and topics of discussion

1. What do you know about bariatric surgery?

This question goes straight to the heart of the matter. Does the trainer understand not only the procedure but also all the restrictions that go along with it? I've heard many stories from clients telling me they hired a personal trainer who always pushed larger calorie intake and advised more carbs and veggies at the expense of protein. They just didn't understand the tool, its limitations, or the protein needs of people who'd had bariatric surgery. It can also be that the person you are interviewing has a negative outlook on this procedure, which this question may uncover.

2. What do you know about obese people and obesity?

This is probably the most important question. The answer will show you the trainer's understanding of what you have gone through and where you are now. Even if you've been out of surgery for a while, you might still have that demon mind that tells you lies about who and what you are. If the person you are hiring to help you doesn't understand or minimizes the struggle of obesity, you will be at a disadvantage.

If you are just out of surgery or in a pre-op stage, having your trainer understand both your physical and mental limitations will help. Knowing that they are meeting you where you are now and working with you from there will make you feel more comfortable and confident.

3. Do you work with beginners?

If you are brand new to working out, you want to make sure you find someone who can work with beginners. This is more important—and may be harder—than you may think. Not all personal trainers are well versed in working with beginners. In fact, many trainers specialize in areas of fitness that aren't meant for beginners, so you need to ask.

If they say yes, you may want to follow up with, "What does a beginner routine look like?" Or better yet, ask them to put you through a short workout so you can experience their method firsthand.

- Tell them your history of exercise (or lack of exercise) if they don't ask you.
- Tell the trainer about all limitations and injuries you have, then ask if they are comfortable working with someone who has those limitations, and what kinds of accommodations or adjustments they can make for you.

It's easy to say yes; it's another thing to prove it. Listen to their answer and ask for clarification when you need it. The answers they give you should jive with your doctor's advice or at least make sense to you.

4. Share your activity goals you want to achieve with this weight loss.

Ask them to briefly describe what they have done with other clients who have similar goals. Their answer should give you an idea of what type of plan they have. It will show you if they are just winging it or if they have thought about how they would approach people similar to you. Of course, the generic plan they present to you shouldn't be your program. What you need will probably be different from what someone else needs, even if the situations are similar, but the trainer's outline will show you the path they intend to take with you.

5. Discuss times in the past that you have started a workout program (if ever) and what stopped you.

Share that experience with the trainer you are interviewing. Ask them how they would help prevent you from falling into that trap again. You may not be comfortable with telling a stranger about a weakness like this. But if you can, it's a good way to uncover how they deal with setbacks that plague us all. The real answer is less about what specific plan they propose and more about how they approach it. This is more about the coach's philosophy about the best way to motivate. For some, it's a soft push; for others, it's more like a drill sergeant. This should give you an idea of whether their style will be effective for you. This is also a great way to see their overall approach to training.

In person or virtual

In addition to finding a trainer, you'll want to know if the place they work is a convenient location for you. For many people, if the gym is located more than three miles from their house or work, the frequency of their visits drops significantly. If the location of the gym where your favorite trainer works isn't close to you, ask about an online training option. You will get a lot of the same services and benefits as you would from working with a personal trainer in person. The trainer will build workouts that are specific to your needs and limitations, schedule the workouts, and monitor your consistency. The downside to online personal training is that there is still a big opportunity to ignore workouts or do less than you need when you are on your own. If you need to have someone in person to keep you on track, then this may not be the best option for you. Yet even this can be mitigated with scheduling a one-on-one session with one of many video meeting apps.

How long should you plan to work with a personal trainer?

It is difficult to know how long you should work with a trainer, but if you are truly just starting out with exercise, I would estimate a minimum of six to nine months. It takes a while to see improvements, and your body will be going through significant changes, which will affect what you can do. Two big changes you'll see: a larger freedom of movement and the ability to do more things. Yet the ability to do more movements and the confidence to do them aren't the same thing.

An example of this came from a client I had early in my career. She taught me a lot about this hesitation of movement due to her presurgery weight. When I started working with Donna, she was about three months out from her gastric bypass and had lost around 50 pounds. Her goal at that time was to slow the muscle mass loss and feel better with movement. One of the exercises I was having her do was a reverse lunge while holding on to the back of a chair for support. It was a movement she could do, and she knew she could do it. But every time she started this exercise, there was a bit of hesitation since this movement used to cause her knees to hurt due to her weight. From a physiological standpoint, this was no longer true, but she needed me there to coach her through the hesitation (and help to keep her form right) to break her fear. She told me later that her mastery of that one movement increased her overall confidence in movement. Having a professional for that one thing went a long way in making the fitness aspect of her journey easier. Having a personal trainer in this first year, one who understands these changes you'll experience and can coach you through any hesitation around some movements, will go a long way to building the confidence of movement.

Pricing

As with any specialist, you are paying for a trainer's experience, not the number of hours each month they train you. At the time of writing, you should expect to pay between $65 and $100-plus per hour for a highly qualified trainer. So taking time to find someone who fits your needs is very important. If you are unable to afford a trainer for all your workouts, ask them if they have other options that will keep you on track. These could be online training, monthly check-ins, and small group classes, or see if they will work with you and a friend to split the cost.

Setting Up a Fitness Plan after Getting Cleared for Exercise

If hiring a personal trainer isn't in the cards for you for whatever reason, then you will need to build your own workout program. This method can be a bit of work to put together, especially if you've never done it before. But once you have a program set up, all it takes to keep it going are some small modifications as you progress.

I've found the best way to build a program is to ask a series of common questions. This way, you'll understand why you are building the program the way you are. It will also help you know how to make modifications as you progress. Note that the following example plan and advice are focused on someone who is new to exercise and has been cleared by their surgeon and primary care doctor to start working out. For some people, the suggestions in this plan may feel limited and easy, and others might find it challenging. Either way, I suggest trying a version of this plan for at least a few weeks. You may feel surprised at how your body reacts.

Q: How long do I need to work out when I start?

A: When you are starting to exercise after you get cleared by your surgeon, make your workout sessions short, about thirty minutes for your strength training and thirty to forty-five minutes for the cardiovascular (cardio) work. These shorter sessions are a good way to gauge how much energy has returned after your surgery. You may be surprised at how quickly you fatigue in the first few sessions. Also, if working out is something you're not really excited about, starting with a shorter session can make it less intimidating. And by ending sooner, you will feel more successful, giving you the motivation to do future sessions. As you continue with these shorter sessions, you will start to become more accustomed to the work. When you notice this, increase the amount of time for your session by about fifteen minutes. Your goal is to be able to do an hour of strength training two or three times a week and four to six hours a week of cardio work.

Your body won't adapt to cardio and strength sessions at the same rate. You'll probably notice that you improve more quickly with your cardio sessions than with your strength training. That's partly because the walking you've been doing has already helped you and partly because your heart and lungs get stronger faster than muscles building strength. So there is a good chance you will see your cardio sessions increase much faster than your strength sessions.

Q: What exercises should I do?

A: For your strength training sessions, focus on basic movements: push, pull, and squat/leg. You can start with machines if you are going to a gym, or resistance bands and body weight if you are working out from home. There are plenty of exercises you can do with those three movements, but if you start with the following exercises, you will be doing well:

- Chest press
- Chest fly
- Lat pulldowns
- Close-grip rows
- Squat or leg press
- Leg extensions
- Leg curls
- Woodchops
- Stability ball crunches

These exercises are all easy to do, and you can use either the machine dedicated to these exercises if you are in a gym or a few resistance bands for your at-home workouts. In either case, you should be able to find some good demonstration videos online.

188

Q: What should I do for cardio exercises?

A: When it comes to adding cardiovascular training into your program, you have two choices: long slow distance training (LSDT) or high-intensity training (HIT). Both have their place in your program, yet knowing when and why to add them is important. Both modes of exercise work off different levels of intensity, so knowing your level of exertion can help you distinguish between them.

Rate of perceived exertion. There are a few ways to judge your level of exertion. One of the easiest is the rate of perceived exertion (RPE). This uses a scale between 0 and 10, where 0 is no exertion and 10 is all out. Most of your work will be somewhere between these two extremes. How you judge where on the scale you land while you are doing work is subjective and different for everyone. Yet once you dial this in, it is shown to be just as effective as heart rate monitors.[61] And in some cases, using this method can improve your overall results versus heart rate monitoring.[61]

Long slow distance training (LSDT). Just as the name suggests, this cardio training doesn't spike your heart rate or leave you gasping for breath. Yet it can be a bit of a misnomer to call it slow. A better name may be long moderate-intensity distance training, with your exertion level being between 5 and 7. At this level, you should be able to train for forty-five minutes or longer. The purpose of LSDT is to build up your muscular endurance (both skeletal and cardiovascular), making it easy to move for thirty minutes to a few hours or more.

When it comes to programming your workouts, start with this type of training. It's much easier on your joints as well as much more approachable. As with strength training, you will need to keep challenging yourself if you want to keep your body improving.

High-intensity training (HIT). This type of cardio training is the opposite of LSDT. With HIT, you will cycle between a high and low heart rate, peaking around at 8 or 9 RPE and recovering to a 6 or 7. Typically, these sessions last no longer than thirty minutes. The purpose of this type of training is to improve your heart rate recovery along with increasing your ability to lose both subcutaneous and visceral fat.[62] For most people who are just starting out, these types of cardio sessions can be very challenging, especially if you have weight-related joint pain. If this is the case, don't plan on putting HIT into your program for at least six months or more post-op. And when you do, start slowly with only one time per week. After a month or so, you can add another day. There is also no need to do HIT more than three days per week to benefit from this type of training.

To see how you can add both types of cardio into your program, refer to the question "What should my schedule look like?" as a good starting point.

Q: What format should I use when I work out?

A: It really doesn't matter what workout format you use, as long as you are working out.

If you're doing strength training in a gym, the best format is the classic reps and sets. That means you'll do one exercise for x number of repetitions (reps), rest for x seconds, and repeat until you've completed all the sets. For example, you might repeat eight chest presses for one set. Then you'd put the weights down, relax your muscles for a minute, then go back and do eight more reps on your second set. If your gym is busy, this lets you take up less space and equipment. But if equipment resources and space are not an issue, you can do a circuit style of training where you set up three or more exercises in a row. You'd do one set of each—maybe eight chest presses, eight squats, and

190

eight jumping jacks. Then you'd take a short rest and do another circuit. These two options have some differences. The classic setup is built around sets and rest intervals, while the circuit format may or may not have rest intervals between exercises. Also take into account your focus. If you are a "one thing at a time" person, the focus of sets and reps will work best for you. If you need variety, then the circuit style may be a better choice.

Q: Where should I start with reps and sets?

A: Start with higher reps using light weights. If you are new to strength training, working with lighter weights gives you the chance to make sure you're doing the movements with the right form. Proper form reduces your chance of injury and maximizes your workout. Also, starting with higher reps will help build more endurance in your muscles, giving you the ability to work out longer. There is more information on how to choose the right weight in the answer to the next question.

Do one to three sets of each exercise for twelve to fifteen reps. If you are brand-new to strength training, then start with just a single set of twelve to fifteen reps. You'll be introducing these movements and resistance to your body while minimizing the soreness that comes from just starting out. Starting more conservatively with your workouts can give you the chance to see how your body will respond to it.

Q: What weight should I start with?

A: When you start lifting, choose a weight related to the number of reps you will be doing. If you're doing fewer reps, start with a slightly heavier weight. So if you plan to do ten reps of a movement, start with a weight that's a little heavier than you'd choose for twenty reps. It's better to start lighter and work your way up to heavier weights if you need. (If you're nervous about using weights, just do the motions without them at first, then use the lightest weight you can find. Next, do the exercise with the weight you chose.) You'll know you've found the right weight for the exercise and repetition range when the final two reps are difficult, but you can still do them with good form. You'll need to do this for each exercise—but it's a one-time process.

Here's an example of how this method works. You're planning three sets of fifteen reps. Pick up a weight that feels easy. Do the fifteen reps. If the final two reps were easy to complete, then on your next set, try a slightly heavier weight for the fifteen reps. If that's easy, add a little more for set three. If you find that difficult but doable for the last two reps, that's the weight you should use next time you're in the gym. If it's still easy, try a slightly heavier one the next time you work out.

The downside to this process is that you can wear yourself out trying to find the right weight. If you're having a difficult time with this, remember it's okay to take your time and extend the process over a few sessions. You'll only go through this process once; when you feel the weight is easy, you can just bump it up a little more.

Speaking of that, you won't stay at this weight, number of repetitions, number of sets, and time working out forever. To keep changing these variables so you can keep building muscle and improving your weight loss, you need to add weight, reps, and even the exercises you do. There are a few ways to do this, explained in the answer to the next question.

Q: When do I change things up?

A: If you are consistent with your workouts, a few months after you start working out, your body will have adapted to the work you are doing. When this starts to happen, you will need to make some changes to your weekly schedule. There are many options to choose from in order to add more time to your strength sessions. To keep it simple, let's just look at two of the most common changes people make: adding more sets and adding more reps. Both will change how much weight you use for an exercise.

As mentioned, when you're new to strength training, fewer sets with lighter weights is a good place to start. Somewhere between one and three sets should be enough. But as your strength grows, the weights will feel lighter, and you may feel like you could use more of a challenge. One way to do this is by adding an extra set to a few of your exercises. These extra sets will add more intensity, fatiguing your muscles a bit more. This will, in turn, get them to build new muscle to compensate for this change. Adding a new set can be a bit much at first, so start with just a few of the exercises in your program. But you can't just keep adding sets—doing a dozen sets, for example, won't cause much more muscle gain.

You can also change the number of reps you complete for each set of the exercises. If you have been doing twelve to fifteen reps for all your exercises, consider dropping that number to ten to twelve reps. When you make this change, you'll notice that the weights you've been using are not very challenging. You'll need to up your resistance to compensate for the lower number of reps—try a heavier weight with the lower number of reps and remember to keep your form. I talked about this more in the previous section on finding your right weight.

Don't make these changes at random times; they should be planned in advance in your program. Here is an example of a yearlong program that uses changes in sets and repetitions over the course of that time.

Months 1 to 3

Sets: 3
Repetitions: 12–15 for each exercise

Months 4 to 6
Sets: 3
Repetitions: 10–12 for each exercise

Months 7 to 9
Sets: 4–5
Repetitions: 10–12 for each exercise

Months 10 to 12
Sets: 5–8
Repetitions: 8–10 for each exercise

This is just one example of what a program could look like. Your program should be based on your goals for strength training and will probably be different. A note about increasing the amount of weight: You'll want to increase the weight by *at most* 10 percent. You may find that this increase puts you between the available resistance. If the increase in weight is less than 5 pounds to the next heavier weight, start with the heavier one, do as many reps as you can with that weight while keeping good form, and then drop back down to the original resistance you were using. Continue with this format for a few weeks until you are able to complete the number of reps and sets for your program with the heavier weight.

Q: What should my schedule look like?

A: Below is a generic example of a six-month program that is set up for someone who has just been cleared for exercise and doesn't have much history with exercise. This program is built to show you what a workout program could look like. Depending on your individual

194

needs and limitations, this program as it is may not work for you.

Something you will notice about this program is the last week of each month is lighter than the other three weeks. This is on purpose to give your body a bit of a rest before you push yourself in the next month.

In months one and two, the sessions are light with two thirty-minute strength sessions, forty-five minutes of cardio (probably walking), light stretching, and two days off. In month three, the cardio starts to push your time; your energy level will determine whether you make this change at this time. Some people are ready for an hour or more of cardio by now; others may lag. Listen to your body and do what you can.

In month four, if you have been consistent with your workouts till this point, there are some changes that happen. First, your program has you doing three hours of strength training each week. Your cardio days are now an hour each, and one day a week is HIT. It's also time to change up your program. Go back to the "When do I change things up?" question to see how that can be done.

Month five is when you add a cardio day on Saturday, bringing you to the 5.5 hours a week of moderate to intense physical activity set up in the guidelines. Also, in week nineteen, both of your weekday cardio sessions are HIT. If this feels a bit aggressive for you, replace one or two of these sessions with an LSDT session. As you start to get stronger, consider adding the HIT sessions back into your program.

Month 6 is where you should be for the remainder of your program. You will see you are down to one day off. The HIT sessions are mixed in with your longer cardio sessions. Yet if you have an activity you want to pursue, then how you program in your cardio will change according to your needs. Also, you may want to make a change to your strength training program at this point.

Finally, you may notice that you're feeling a bit fatigued physically and mentally at the six-month mark. That's to be expected; your body is telling you 'you need a break', so take it. Build month seven to be a lighter-than-normal month, dropping back down to what you did in month three. By doing this, you are reducing your chance of future injury as well as setting yourself up for bigger gains in future sessions.

6 Month Example Workout Schedule

Month 1	Sun	Mon	Tues	Wed	Thurs	Fri	Sat
Week 1	Off	30 min. strength	45 min. cardio	30 min. strength	45 min. cardio	Stretch /Yoga	Off
Week 2	Off	30 min strength	45 min. cardio	30 min. strength	45 min. cardio	Stretch /Yoga	Off
Week 3	Off	30 min strength	45 min. cardio	30 min. strength	45 min. cardio	Stretch /Yoga	Off
Week 4	Off	30 min strength	Off	30 min. strength	30 min. cardio	Stretch /Yoga	Off
Month 2	Sun	Mon	Tues	Wed	Thurs	Fri	Sat
Week 5	Off	45 min Strength	30 min cardio	45 min Strength	30 min cardio	Stretch /Yoga	Off
Week 6	Off	45 min Strength	45 min. cardio	45 min Strength	45 min. cardio	Stretch /Yoga	Off
Week 7	Off	45 min Strength	45 min. cardio	45 min Strength	45 min. cardio	Stretch /Yoga	Off
Week 8	Off	30 min Strength	45 min. cardio	30 min Strength	45 min. cardio	Stretch /Yoga	Off
Month 3	Sun	Mon	Tues	Wed	Thurs	Fri	Sat
Week 9	Off	60 min Strength	30 min cardio	60 min Strength	30 min cardio	Stretch /Yoga	Off

	Sun	Mon	Tues	Wed	Thurs	Fri	Sat
Week 10	Off	60 min Strength	45-60 min cardio	60 min Strength	45-60 min cardio	Stretch /Yoga	Off
Week 11	Off	60 min Strength	45-60 min cardio	60 min Strength	45-60 min cardio	Stretch /Yoga	Off
Week 12	Off	45 min Strength	45 min. cardio	45 min Strength	Stretch /Yoga	Stretch /Yoga	Off
Month 4	Sun	Mon	Tues	Wed	Thurs	Fri	Sat
Week 13	Off	60 min Strength	45-60 min cardio	60 min Strength	45-60 min cardio	60 min Strength	Off
Week 14	Off	60 min Strength	60 min cardio	60 min Strength	60 min cardio	60 min Strength	Off
Week 15	Off	60 min Strength	30 min HIT	60 min Strength	60 min cardio	60 min Strength	Off
Week 16	Off	60 min Strength	30 min HIT	45 min Strength	Stretch /Yoga	60 min Strength	Off
Month 5	Sun	Mon	Tues	Wed	Thurs	Fri	Sat
Week 17	Off	60 min Strength	30 min HIT	60 min Strength	60 min cardio	60 min Strength	60 min cardio
Week 18	Off	60 min Strength	30 min HIT	60 min Strength	60 min cardio	60 min Strength	60 min cardio
Week 19	Off	60 min Strength	30 min HIT	60 min Strength	30 min HIT	60 min Strength	60 min cardio
Week 20	Off	60 min Strength	45-60 min cardio	45 min Strength	Stretch /Yoga	60 min Strength	Off
Month 6	Sun	Mon	Tues	Wed	Thurs	Fri	Sat

Week 21	Off	60 min Strength	30 min HIT	60 min Strength	30 min HIT	60 min Strength	30 min HIIT
Week 22	Off	60 min Strength	60 min cardio	60 min Strength	60 min cardio	60 min Strength	60 min cardio
Week 23	Off	60 min Strength	30 min HIT	60 min Strength	30 min HIT	60 min Strength	30 min HIIT
Week 24	Off	60 min Strength	60 min cardio	45 min Strength	60 min cardio	60 min Strength	60 min cardio

References

1. Johnson RJ, Johnson BL, Blackhurst DW, Bour ES, Cobb WS Iv, Carbonell AM II, et al. Bariatric surgery is associated with a reduced risk of mortality in morbidly obese patients with a history of major cardiovascular events. Am Surg [Internet]. 2012;78(6):685–92. Available from: http://dx.doi.org/10.1177/000313481207800623

2. Riebl SK, Davy BM. The hydration equation: Update on water balance and cognitive performance: Update on water balance and cognitive performance. ACSMs Health Fit J [Internet]. 2013;17(6):21–8. Available from: http://dx.doi.org/10.1249/FIT.0b013e3182a9570f

3. Study suggests weight-loss surgery may release toxic compounds from fat into the bloodstream. Johns Hopkins Bloomberg School of Public Health. 2021. Available from: https://www.jhsph.edu/news/news-releases/2019/study-suggests-weight-loss-surgery-may-release-toxic-compounds-from-fat-into-the-bloodstream.html

4. Fénichel P, Coquillard P, Brucker-Davis F, Marchand P, Cano-Sancho G, Boda M, et al. Sustained bloodstream release of persistent organic pollutants induced by extensive weight loss after bariatric surgery: Implications for women of childbearing age. Environ Int.

2021;151(106400):106400. Available from:
https://www.sciencedirect.com/science/article/pii/S0160412021000246

5. Cho E, Chen WY, Hunter DJ, Stampfer MJ, Colditz GA, Hankinson SE, et al. Red meat intake and risk of breast cancer among premenopausal women. Arch Intern Med [Internet]. 2006;166(20):2253–9. Available from:
https://jamanetwork.com/journals/jamainternalmedicine/fullarticle/411256

6. Ferguson LR. Meat and cancer. Meat Sci [Internet]. 2010;84(2):308–13. Available from:
http://dx.doi.org/10.1016/j.meatsci.2009.06.032

7. Demeyer D, Mertens B, De Smet S, Ulens M. Mechanisms linking colorectal cancer to the consumption of (processed) red meat: A review. Crit Rev Food Sci Nutr [Internet]. 2016;56(16):2747–66. Available from:
http://dx.doi.org/10.1080/10408398.2013.873886

8. Livhits M, Mercado C, Yermilov I, Parikh JA, Dutson E, Mehran A, et al. Is social support associated with greater weight loss after bariatric surgery?: a systematic review: Social support and bariatric surgery. Obes Rev [Internet]. 2011;12(2):142–8. Available from:
https://www.ncbi.nlm.nih.gov/books/NBK81240/

9. Orth WS, Madan AK, Taddeucci RJ, Coday M, Tichansky DS. Support group meeting attendance is associated with better weight loss. Obes Surg [Internet]. 2008;18(4):391–4. Available from: http://dx.doi.org/10.1007/s11695-008-9444-8

10. Song Z, Reinhardt K, Buzdon M, Liao P. Association between support group attendance and weight loss after Roux-en-Y gastric bypass. Surg Obes Relat Dis [Internet]. 2008;4(2):100–3. Available from: http://dx.doi.org/10.1016/j.soard.2007.02.010

11. Elakkary E, Elhorr A, Aziz F, Gazayerli M, Silva Y. Do support groups play a role in weight loss after laparoscopic adjustable gastric banding? Obes Surg [Internet]. 2006;16(3):331–4. Available from: http://dx.doi.org/10.1381/096089206776116499

12. Hildebrandt SE. Effects of participation in bariatric support group after roux-en-Y gastric bypass. Obes Surg [Internet]. 1998;8(5):535–42. Available from: http://dx.doi.org/10.1381/096089298765554115

13. Beck NN, Johannsen M, Støving RK, Mehlsen M, Zachariae R. Do postoperative psychotherapeutic interventions and support groups influence weight loss following bariatric surgery? A systematic review and meta-analysis of randomized and nonrandomized trials. Obes Surg [Internet]. 2012;22(11):1790–7. Available from: http://dx.doi.org/10.1007/s11695-012-0739-4

14. Ahmed K, Penney N, Darzi A, Purkayastha S. Taste changes after bariatric surgery: A systematic review. Obes Surg. 2018;28(10):3321–32. Available from: http://dx.doi.org/10.1007/s11695-018-3420-8

15. Holinski F, Menenakos C, Haber G, Olze H, Ordemann J. Olfactory and gustatory function after bariatric surgery. Obes Surg [Internet]. 2015 ;25(12):2314–20. Available from: https://pubmed.ncbi.nlm.nih.gov/25910980/

16. Nehlig A. Effects of coffee on the Gastro-intestinal tract: A narrative review and literature update. Nutrients. 2022;14(2):399. Available from: http://dx.doi.org/10.3390/nu14020399

17. Eweis DS, Abed F, Stiban J. Carbon dioxide in carbonated beverages induces ghrelin release and increased food consumption in male rats: Implications on the onset of obesity. Obes Res Clin Pract. 2017;11(5):534–43. Available from: http://dx.doi.org/10.1016/j.orcp.2017.02.001

18. Shiffman ML, Sugerman HJ, Kellum JH, Brewer WH, Moore EW. Gallstones in patients with morbid obesity. Relationship to body weight, weight loss and gallbladder bile cholesterol solubility. Int J Obes Relat Metab Disord. 1993;17(3):153–8. Available from: https://europepmc.org/article/med/8385075

19. Egberts K, Brown WA, Brennan L, O'Brien PE. Does exercise improve weight loss after bariatric surgery? A systematic review. Obes Surg. 2012;22(2):335–41. Available from: http://dx.doi.org/10.1007/s11695-011-0544-5

20. Bond DS, Phelan S, Wolfe LG, Evans RK, Meador JG, Kellum JM, et al. Becoming physically active after bariatric surgery is associated with improved weight loss and health-related quality of life. Obesity (Silver Spring). 2009;17(1):78–83. Available from: http://dx.doi.org/10.1038/oby.2008.501

21. Metcalf B, Rabkin RA, Rabkin JM, Metcalf LJ, Lehman-Becker LB. Weight loss composition: The effects of exercise following obesity surgery as measured by bioelectrical impedance analysis. Obes Surg. 2005;15(2):183–6. Available from: http://dx.doi.org/10.1381/0960892053268381

22. Paluska SA, Schwenk TL. Physical activity and mental health: Current concepts. Sports Med. 2000;29(3):167–80. Available from: http://dx.doi.org/10.2165/00007256-200029030-00003

23. Silveira H, Moraes H, Oliveira N, Coutinho ESF, Laks J, Deslandes A. Physical exercise and clinically depressed patients: a systematic review

and meta-analysis. Neuropsychobiology. 2013;67(2):61–8. Available from: https://pubmed.ncbi.nlm.nih.gov/23295766/

24. Joo J, Williamson SA, Vazquez AI, Fernandez JR, Bray MS. The influence of 15-week exercise training on dietary patterns among young adults. Int J Obes (Lond). 2019;43(9):1681–90. Available from: http://dx.doi.org/10.1038/s41366-018-0299-3

25. Wouters EJ, Larsen JK, Zijlstra H, van Ramshorst B, Geenen R. Physical activity after surgery for severe obesity: The role of exercise cognitions. Obes Surg. 2011;21(12):1894–9. Available from: http://dx.doi.org/10.1007/s11695-010-0276-y

26. Morales-Marroquin E, Kohl HW 3rd, Knell G, de la Cruz-Muñoz N, Messiah SE. Resistance training in post-metabolic and bariatric surgery patients: A systematic review. Obes Surg [Internet]. 2020 ;30(10):4071–80. Available from: https://pubmed.ncbi.nlm.nih.gov/32671727/

27. Laviada-Molina H, Molina-Segui F, Pérez-Gaxiola G, Cuello-García C, Arjona-Villicaña R, Espinosa-Marrón A, et al. Effects of nonnutritive sweeteners on body weight and BMI in diverse clinical contexts: Systematic review and meta-analysis. Obes Rev [Internet]. 2020;21(7). Available from: http://dx.doi.org/10.1111/obr.13020

205

28. Fowler SP, Williams K, Resendez RG, Hunt KJ, Hazuda HP, Stern MP. Fueling the obesity epidemic? Artificially sweetened beverage use and long-term weight gain. Obesity (Silver Spring) [Internet]. 2008;16(8):1894–900. Available from: http://dx.doi.org/10.1038/oby.2008.284

29. Bleich SN, Wolfson JA, Vine S, Wang YC. Diet-beverage consumption and caloric intake among US adults, overall and by body weight. Am J Public Health [Internet]. 2014;104(3):e72–8. Available from: http://dx.doi.org/10.2105/ajph.2013.301556

30. Hagedorn JC, Encarnacion B, Brat GA, Morton JM. Does gastric bypass alter alcohol metabolism? Surg Obes Relat Dis [Internet]. 2007;3(5):543–8. Available from: http://dx.doi.org/10.1016/j.soard.2007.07.003

31. Svensson P-A, Anveden Å, Romeo S, Peltonen M, Ahlin S, Burza MA, et al. Alcohol consumption and alcohol problems after bariatric surgery in the swedish obese subjects study: Alcohol Consumption and Alcohol Problems After Bariatric Surgery. Obesity (Silver Spring) [Internet]. 2013;21(12):2444–51. Available from: http://dx.doi.org/10.1002/oby.20397

32. King WC, Chen J-Y, Mitchell JE, Kalarchian MA, Steffen KJ, Engel SG, et al. Prevalence of alcohol use disorders before and after bariatric surgery. JAMA [Internet]. 2012;307(23). Available from:

http://dx.doi.org/10.1001/jama.2012.6147

33. Alcohol use and health risks: Survey results
[Internet]. Bariatrictimes.com.. Available from:
https://bariatrictimes.com/alcohol-use-and-health-
risks-survey-results/

34. Ostlund MP, Backman O, Marsk R, Stockeld D,
Lagergren J, Rasmussen F, et al. Increased
admission for alcohol dependence after gastric
bypass surgery compared with restrictive bariatric
surgery. JAMA Surg [Internet]. 2013;148(4):374–7.
Available from:
https://jamanetwork.com/journals/jamasurgery/fullar
ticle/1679649

35. Pedram P, Wadden D, Amini P, Gulliver W, Randell
E, Cahill F, et al. Food addiction: Its prevalence and
significant association with obesity in the general
population. PLoS One [Internet]. 2013;8(9):e74832.
Available from:
http://dx.doi.org/10.1371/journal.pone.0074832

36. Lerma-Cabrera JM, Carvajal F, Lopez-Legarrea P.
Food addiction as a new piece of the obesity
framework. Nutr J [Internet]. 2015;15(1). Available
from: http://dx.doi.org/10.1186/s12937-016-0124-6

37. Chiappetta S, Stier C, Hadid MA, Malo N,
Theodoridou S, Weiner R, et al. Remission of food
addiction does not induce cross-addiction after

sleeve gastrectomy and gastric bypass: A prospective cohort study. Obes Facts [Internet]. 2020;13(3):307–20. Available from: http://dx.doi.org/10.1159/000506838

38. What is addiction transfer? [Internet]. Modern Network. 2022]. Available from: https://www.springboardrecovery.com/understandin g-addiction-transfer/

39. Grossman E, Grossman A, Schein MH, Zimlichman R, Gavish B. Breathing-control lowers blood pressure. J Hum Hypertens [Internet]. 2001;15(4):263–9. Available from: http://dx.doi.org/10.1038/sj.jhh.1001147

40. Rasheed H, Mahgoub D, Hegazy R, El-Komy M, Abdel Hay R, Hamid MA, et al. Serum ferritin and vitamin D in female hair loss: Do they play a role? Skin Pharmacol Physiol [Internet]. 2013;26(2):101–7. Available from: http://dx.doi.org/10.1159/000346698

41. Moeinvaziri M, Mansoori P, Holakooee K, Safaee Naraghi Z, Abbasi A. Iron status in diffuse telogen hair loss among women. Acta Dermatovenerol Croat [Internet]. 2009 ;17(4):279–84. Available from: https://pubmed.ncbi.nlm.nih.gov/20021982/

42. Almohanna HM, Ahmed AA, Tsatalis JP, Tosti A. The role of vitamins and minerals in hair loss: A

review. Dermatol Ther (Heidelb) [Internet].
2019;9(1):51–70. Available from:
http://dx.doi.org/10.1007/s13555-018-0278-6

43. Harrison S, Sinclair R. Telogen effluvium: Telogen
effluvium. Clin Exp Dermatol [Internet]. 2002
;27(5):389–385. Available from:
https://pubmed.ncbi.nlm.nih.gov/12190639/

44. Rushton DH, Dover R, Norris MJ. Is there really no
clear association between low serum ferritin and
chronic diffuse telogen hair loss? Br J Dermatol
[Internet]. 2003 ;148(6):1282–4; author reply 1284.
Available from:
https://pubmed.ncbi.nlm.nih.gov/12828773/

45. Neve HJ, Bhatti WA, Soulsby C, Kincey J, Taylor
TV. Reversal of Hair Loss following Vertical
Gastroplasty when Treated with Zinc Sulphate.
Obes Surg [Internet]. 1996;6(1):63–5. Available
from:
http://dx.doi.org/10.1381/096089296765557295

46. Yavuz IH, Yavuz GO, Bilgili SG, Demir H, Demir C.
Assessment of heavy metal and trace element
levels in patients with telogen effluvium. Indian J
Dermatol [Internet]. 2018 ;63(3):246–50. Available
from: https://pubmed.ncbi.nlm.nih.gov/29937562/

47. Biörserud C, Olbers T, Søvik TT, Mala T, Elander A,
Olsén MF. Experience of excess skin after gastric

bypass or duodenal switch in patients with super obesity. Surg Obes Relat Dis [Internet]. 2014];10(5):891–6. Available from: https://pubmed.ncbi.nlm.nih.gov/24837559/

48. Halawi A, Abiad F, Abbas O. Bariatric surgery and its effects on the skin and skin diseases. Obes Surg [Internet]. 2013;23(3):408–13. Available from: http://dx.doi.org/10.1007/s11695-012-0859-x

49. Geliebter A, Schachter S, Lohmann-Walter C, Feldman H, Hashim SA. Reduced stomach capacity in obese subjects after dieting. Am J Clin Nutr [Internet]. 1996;63(2):170–3. Available from: http://dx.doi.org/10.1093/ajcn/63.2.170

50. Applegate KL, Friedman KE. The impact of weight loss surgery on romantic relationships. Bariatr Nurs Surg Patient Care [Internet]. 2008;3(2):135–41. Available from: http://dx.doi.org/10.1089/bar.2008.9976

51. Hemmingsson E, Johansson K, Reynisdottir S. Effects of childhood abuse on adult obesity: a systematic review and meta-analysis: Childhood abuse and adult obesity. Obes Rev [Internet]. 2014;15(11):882–93. Available from: https://pubmed.ncbi.nlm.nih.gov/25123205/

52. Felitti VJ, Anda RF, Nordenberg D, Williamson DF, Spitz AM, Edwards V, et al. Relationship of

childhood abuse and household dysfunction to many of the leading causes of death in adults. The Adverse Childhood Experiences (ACE) Study. Am J Prev Med [Internet]. 1998 ;14(4):245–58. Available from: https://pubmed.ncbi.nlm.nih.gov/9635069/

53. Weiner EJ, Stephens L. Sexual barrier weight: A new approach. Eat Disord [Internet]. 1993;1(3–4):241–9. Available from: http://dx.doi.org/10.1080/10640269308251163

54. Teitelman M, Grotegut C, Williams N, Lewis J. The impact of bariatric surgery on menstrual patterns. Obes Surg [Internet]. 2006;16(11):1457–63. Available from: http://dx.doi.org/10.1381/096089206778870148

55. Escobar-Morreale HF, Botella-Carretero JI, Álvarez-Blasco F, Sancho J, San Millán JL. The polycystic ovary syndrome associated with morbid obesity may resolve after weight loss induced by bariatric surgery. J Clin Endocrinol Metab [Internet]. 2005;90(12):6364–9. Available from: http://dx.doi.org/10.1210/jc.2005-1490

56. Sussman D, van Eede M, Wong MD, Adamson SL, Henkelman M. Effects of a ketogenic diet during pregnancy on embryonic growth in the mouse. BMC Pregnancy Childbirth [Internet]. 2013;13(1). Available from: http://dx.doi.org/10.1186/1471-2393-13-109

57. Hammoud A, Gibson M, Hunt SC, Adams TD, Carrell DT, Kolotkin RL, et al. Effect of Roux-en-Y gastric bypass surgery on the sex steroids and Quality of Life in obese men. J Clin Endocrinol Metab [Internet]. 2009;94(4):1329–32. Available from: http://dx.doi.org/10.1210/jc.2008-1598

58. di Frega AS, Dale B, Di Matteo L, Wilding M. Secondary male factor infertility after Roux-en-Y gastric bypass for morbid obesity: Case report. Hum Reprod [Internet]. 2005;20(4):997–8. Available from: http://dx.doi.org/10.1093/humrep/deh707

59. Freire RH, Borges MC, Alvarez-Leite JI, Correia MITD. Food quality, physical activity, and nutritional follow-up as determinant of weight regain after Roux-en-Y gastric bypass. Nutrition [Internet]. 2012;28(1):53–8. Available from: http://dx.doi.org/10.1016/j.nut.2011.01.011

60. Nymo S, Lundanes J, Aukan M, Sandvik J, Johnsen G, Græslie H, et al. Diet and physical activity are associated with suboptimal weight loss and weight regain 10–15 years after Roux-en-Y gastric bypass: A cross-sectional study. Obes Res Clin Pract [Internet]. 2022;16(2):163–9. Available from: http://dx.doi.org/10.1016/j.orcp.2022.03.006

61. Koltyn, K. F. and Morgan, W. P. (1992) "Efficacy of perceptual versus heart rate monitoring in the

development of endurance," British journal of sports medicine, 26(2), pp. 132–134. doi: 10.1136/bjsm.26.2.132.

62. Boutcher, S. H. (2011). High-intensity intermittent exercise and fat loss. *Journal of Obesity*, *2011*, 1–10. https://doi.org/10.1155/2011/868305